Gastrointestinal Imaging

A Teaching File

Gastrointestinal Imaging

A Teaching File

Editors

Courtney Coursey Moreno, MD
Assistant Professor of Radiology
Director of Ultrasound
Department of Radiology and Imaging Sciences
Emory University School of Medicine
Atlanta, Georgia

Pardeep Kumar Mittal, MD
Assistant Professor of Radiology
Director of MRI Body Imaging
Department of Radiology and Imaging Sciences
Emory University School of Medicine
Atlanta, Georgia

Wolters Kluwer
Health
Philadelphia · Baltimore · New York · London
Buenos Aires · Hong Kong · Sydney · Tokyo

Senior Executive Editor: Jonathan W. Pine, Jr.
Acquisitions Editor: Ryan Shaw
Product Development Editor: Amy G. Dinkel
Product Production Manager: David Orzechowski
Senior Manufacturing Coordinator: Beth Welsh
Marketing Manager: Dan Dressler
Senior Designer: Stephen Druding
Production Service: Integra Software Services Pvt. Ltd.

Printed in China

Library of Congress Cataloging-in-Publication Data

Gastrointestinal imaging (Moreno)
 Gastrointestinal imaging : a teaching file / editors, Courtney Coursey Moreno,
Pardeep Kumar Mittal.
  p. ; cm.
 Includes bibliographical references and index.
 ISBN 978-1-4511-7337-6
 ISBN 1-4511-7337-7
 I. Moreno, Courtney Coursey, editor of compilation.   II. Mittal, Pardeep Kumar, editor of compilation.   III. Title.
 [DNLM: 1. Digestive System Diseases—diagnosis—Case Reports.   2. Diagnosis, Differential—Case Reports.   3. Diagnostic Imaging—methods—Case Reports. WI 141]
 RC804.D52
 616.3'30754—dc23

                                                2014003469

Care has been taken to confirm the accuracy of the information presented and to describe generally accepted practices. However, the authors, editors, and publisher are not responsible for errors or omissions or for any consequences from application of the information in this book and make no warranty, expressed or implied, with respect to the currency, completeness, or accuracy of the contents of the publication. Application of the information in a particular situation remains the professional responsibility of the practitioner.

The authors, editors, and publisher have exerted every effort to ensure that drug selection and dosage set forth in this text are in accordance with current recommendations and practice at the time of publication. However, in view of ongoing research, changes in government regulations, and the constant flow of information relating to drug therapy and drug reactions, the reader is urged to check the package insert for each drug for any change in indications and dosage and for added warnings and precautions. This is particularly important when the recommended agent is a new or infrequently employed drug.

Some drugs and medical devices presented in the publication have Food and Drug Administration (FDA) clearance for limited use in restricted research settings. It is the responsibility of the health care provider to ascertain the FDA status of each drug or device planned for use in their clinical practice.

To purchase additional copies of this book, call our customer service department at (800) 638-3030 or fax orders to (301) 223-2320. International customers should call (301) 223-2300.

Visit Lippincott Williams & Wilkins on the Internet: at LWW.com. Lippincott Williams & Wilkins customer service representatives are available from 8:30 am to 6 pm, EST.

10 9 8 7 6 5 4 3 2 1

To my son, Ricky, who amazes me every day. To my husband, Ricardo, for his support and ideas. To my parents, Martha and Jeff Coursey, for encouraging me to follow my dreams.

Courtney Coursey Moreno

It is with great pleasure that I dedicate this book to my family, mentors, colleagues, residents, fellows, and students for their guidance and contribution in both my personal and professional life.

Pardeep Kumar Mittal

Teaching Files are one of the hallmarks of education in radiology. When there was a need for a comprehensive series to provide the resident and practicing radiologist with the kind of personal consultation with the experts normally found only in the setting of a teaching hospital, Lippincott Williams & Wilkins was proud to have created a series that answers this need.

Actual cases have been culled from extensive teaching files in major medical centers. The discussions presented mimic those performed on a daily basis between residents and faculty members in all radiology departments.

This series is designed so that each case can be studied as an unknown. A consistent format is used to present each case. A brief clinical history is given, followed by several images. Then, relevant findings, differential diagnosis, and final diagnosis are given, followed by a discussion of the case. The authors thereby guide the reader through the interpretation of each case.

This year we've made additional changes to the series. Cases have been randomized to better prepare the reader for the challenges of the clinical setting. In addition, to answer the growing demand for Web-based product, we have included more cases online, which has left us, in turn, able to offer a more cost-effective product.

We hope that this series will continue to be a trusted teaching tool for radiologists at any stage of training or practice, and that it will also be a benefit to clinicians whose patients undergo these imaging studies.

The Publisher

In compiling the cases for this volume, we sought to create a high-value resource for trainees learning the basics of gastrointestinal imaging (fluoroscopy, CT, and MR) and also for those studying for board and certifying examinations. To that end, we have included all of the topics listed at the time of this writing in the Gastrointestinal Imaging section of the publicly available American Board of Radiology Core Exam and Maintenance of Certification study guides.

To round out the 300 cases in this teaching file, we included additional fluoroscopy, CT, and MR cases that we hope you will find interesting and educational.

Cases are grouped into three chapters based on modality so that trainees can use this teaching file efficiently during modality-based rotations.

We hope that you will find this collection of cases to be a helpful resource as you train your eye to recognize findings at fluoroscopy, review the variety of diagnoses that can be made at CT, and get your feet wet with the basics of body MR.

Courtney Coursey Moreno
Pardeep Kumar Mittal

Thank you to Drs. Carl Ravin and Linda Gray Leithe for giving me my start in radiology. Thank you to mentors present and past including Drs. Rendon Nelson, Don Frush, Erik Paulson, Tracy Jaffe, George Bisset, Caroline Hollingsworth, Sal Martinez, John H.M. Austin, Dean Danner, Bill Small, Bill Torres, Deb Baumgarten, and Carolyn Meltzer. Thank you to all of the attendings at Duke who taught me so much during residency and fellowship, with special thanks to those in the abdominal imaging division. Thank you to Deb Baumgarten for sharing the opportunity to complete this project with our division. Thank you to Eric Jablonowski and Kevin Makowski for converting some of the films to digital images for this volume. Thank you to Amy Dinkel and the late Jonathan Pine from Wolters Kluwer for making putting this project together such a pleasant experience.

Courtney Coursey Moreno

Thank you to all of my mentors, past and present, at New York Methodist Hospital in Brooklyn, NY, University of Connecticut Health Center, Medical College of Georgia, and Emory University School of Medicine who helped me when I was a resident in nuclear medicine and diagnostic radiology and during my abdominal imaging fellowship. I also want to thank my staff, mentors, and colleagues at Emory University School of Medicine Department of Radiology and Imaging Sciences for their immense support and guidance. Kevin Makowski and Eric Jablonowski's diligent efforts to convert old hard copy radiographs to digital images were necessary to complete this gastrointestinal teaching file project. Finally, this project would not have been possible without the expert guidance of Amy Dinkel and the late Jonathan Pine from Wolters Kluwer.

Pardeep Kumar Mittal

CHAPTER 1

Fluoroscopy

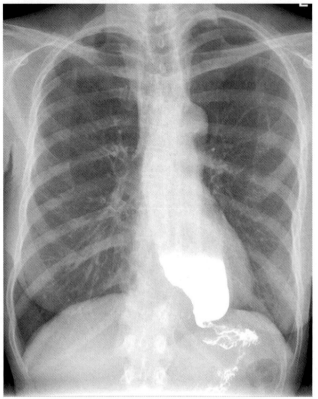

FIGURE 1.1A

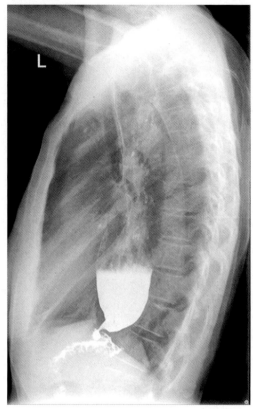

FIGURE 1.1B

FINDINGS Frontal and lateral radiographs (A, B) obtained at the conclusion of a barium swallow demonstrate a dilated, patulous esophagus. Distally, the esophagus is narrowed. At real-time imaging, ingested contrast material appeared to slide down the walls of the esophagus without any real assistance from primary or secondary peristaltic waves. Ingested contrast material pooled in the distal esophagus and eventually slowly emptied into the stomach. At the conclusion of the study, a moderate amount of contrast material remained in the esophagus as seen in these radiographs.

DIFFERENTIAL DIAGNOSIS Achalasia, distal esophageal cancer.

DIAGNOSIS Achalasia.

DISCUSSION Achalasia is a primary esophageal motility disorder characterized by the failure of the lower esophageal sphincter to relax. At barium swallow, the characteristic "bird-beak" or narrowed appearance of the distal esophagus reflects this failure of the distal esophageal sphincter to relax. At initial presentation, all patients in whom achalasia is suspected should undergo upper endoscopy to exclude a distal esophageal mass causing a pseudoachalasia appearance.

Early in the disease process, achalasia may be misdiagnosed as an isolated distal esophageal stricture. As the disease progresses, increasingly impaired peristalsis is noted due to progressively impaired function of neural networks in the smooth muscle of the distal esophagus. Large-volume food debris may be present in the esophagus at the time of barium swallow even if the patient has not consumed any food by mouth for many hours prior to the study.

A variety of treatment options are available for patients with achalasia (see Question 2). At some centers, timed barium swallow is performed as a way to evaluate esophageal clearance pre- and post-treatment. Patients ingest 100 to 200 mL of contrast material (volume ingested should be recorded and repeated in follow-up studies), and upright left posterior oblique images are obtained 1, 2, and 5 minutes post contrast ingestion. The percentage of contrast material cleared at 5 minutes is estimated by comparing the computed area of contrast material (width × height of esophageal contrast column) in the 1- and 5-minute films.

Questions for Further Thought

1. What is the etiology of achalasia?
2. What are current treatment options for achalasia patients?

Reporting Requirements

1. Suggest the diagnosis of achalasia.
2. Recommend esophagogastroduodenoscopy (EGD) at initial presentation to rule out an obstructing mass resulting in pseudoachalasia.

What the Treating Physician Needs to Know

1. At initial presentation, achalasia can be difficult to distinguish from a distal esophageal malignant stricture.
2. At initial presentation, all patients with suspected achalasia based on barium swallow should undergo upper endoscopy to exclude a distal esophageal mass resulting in pseudoachalasia.

Answers

1. The etiology of achalasia is unknown. Theories include a genetic, autoimmune, or infectious trigger that incites an inflammatory process that damages the neural networks in esophageal smooth muscle.
2. At the present time there is no way to reverse the nerve damage that produces achalasia. Current treatments are aimed at relieving symptoms. Myotomy (via open or laparoscopic approach) or endoscopic balloon dilatation may be performed to dilate a distal esophageal stricture. Botulinum toxin injection via endoscopy can relax the lower esophageal sphincter and provide short-term symptom palliation. Medical management including calcium channel blockers or long-acting nitrates can provide short-term symptomatic relief because of their muscle relaxation properties. The last line treatment option for patients with a megaesophagus who do not respond to other treatments is esophagectomy.

REFERENCES

1. de Oliveira JMA, Birgisson S, Doinoff C, et al. Timed barium swallow: a simple technique for evaluating esophageal emptying in patients with achalasia. Am J Roentgenol 1997;169:473-479.
2. Vaezi MF, Richter JE. Diagnosis and management of achalasia. Am J Gastroenterol 1999;94:3406-3412.

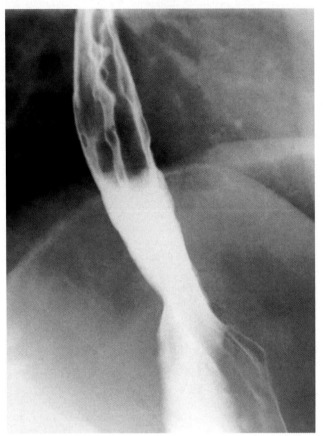

FIGURE 1.2A

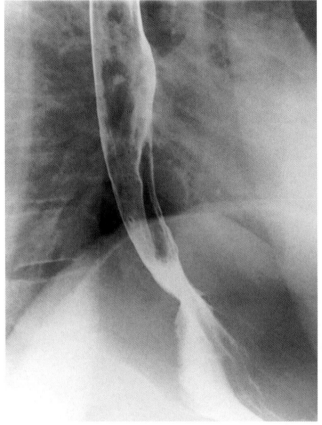

FIGURE 1.2B

FINDINGS Air-contrast barium swallow (A, B) demonstrates linear, tubular filling defects running parallel to the longitudinal axis of the esophagus. These structures were intermittently visible during the barium swallow.

DIFFERENTIAL DIAGNOSIS Normal longitudinal folds, varices, varicoid esophageal cancer.

DIAGNOSIS Varices.

DISCUSSION Esophageal varices are dilated submucosal veins within the wall of the esophagus. Varices most commonly occur in patients with portal hypertension and are prone to bleeding. Bleeding from esophageal varices is the cause of death in approximately one-third of patients with chronic liver disease and portal hypertension.

Esophageal varices are graded based on their appearance at endoscopy. Grade 1 varices are small, straight varices. Grade 2 varices are large, tortuous varices that occupy less than one-third of the esophageal lumen. Grade 3 varices are large, tortuous varices that occupy more than one-third of the lumen.

Fluoroscopy is a relatively insensitive test for the demonstration of varices. Meticulous attention to technique is necessary to demonstrate varices as they may be intermittently visible during barium studies as in the above case. For example, full-column barium may efface varices rendering them invisible. Varices also may change caliber depending on intrathoracic pressure. Placing the patient in a prone, right anterior oblique position can aid in the demonstration of varices by (1) increasing variceal distention due to gravity effects and (2) improving mucosal coating by slowing the transit of barium. Valsalva maneuver may increase the conspicuity of varices. Single small sips of barium may improve detection of varices as repeated peristalsis may efface varices.

Varicoid esophageal cancer is usually more irregular in appearance and a more fixed abnormality when compared with esophageal varices. However, when in doubt contrast-enhanced computed tomography (CT) or magnetic resonance (MR) is a noninvasive way to rule in or rule out most varices.

The collapsed esophagus often demonstrates longitudinal folds. However, these folds generally run the entire length of the esophagus and can be distinguished from varices that are usually isolated to the upper third or lower third of the esophagus (see below).

Questions for Further Thought

1. Define uphill varix.
2. Define downhill varix.

Reporting Requirement

1. Report the presence of probable esophageal varices along the distal esophagus.

What the Treating Physician Needs to Know

1. Endoscopy is the gold standard test for diagnosing and grading varices.
2. CT and MR are more sensitive than barium swallow for the identification of varices.

Answers

1. Uphill varices occur in patients with portal hypertension and are usually confined to the lower third of the esophagus. These collateral pathways allow blood to bypass the liver and return to the heart via enlarged esophageal collateral vessels and the superior vena cava.
2. Downhill varices occur in patients with superior vena cava obstruction and are usually located in the upper third or middle third of the esophagus. These dilated esophageal collateral vessels allow blood to return to the heart via the portal venous system and the inferior vena cava.

REFERENCES

1. Levine MS, Rubesin SE. Diseases of the esophagus: diagnosis with esophagography. Radiology 2005;237:414-427.
2. de Franchis R, Primignani M. Natural history of portal hypertension in patients with cirrhosis. Clin Liver Dis 2001;5:645-663.

CLINICAL HISTORY *52-year-old woman with dysphagia.*

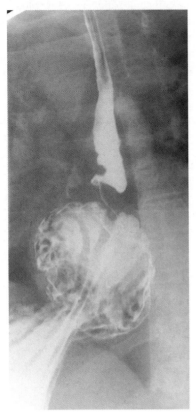

FIGURE 1.3A

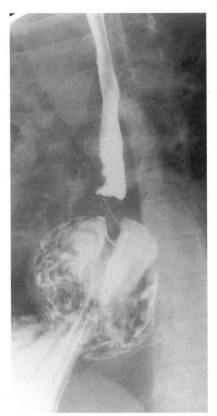

FIGURE 1.3B

FINDINGS Barium swallow (A, B) demonstrates herniation of the gastric rugal folds above the diaphragm.

DIFFERENTIAL DIAGNOSIS Sliding hiatal hernia, paraesophageal hernia.

DIAGNOSIS Sliding hiatal hernia.

DISCUSSION "Hiatus" is defined as an opening and "hernia" is defined as a bulge or protrusion of an organ through a structure that normally contains it. The term "hiatal hernia" is used to describe herniation of the stomach through the esophageal hiatus into the chest.

Since the esophagus must expand and contract to permit the transit of food, the esophagus is not tightly fixed to the diaphragm at the esophageal hiatus. Rather, the phrenoesophageal ligaments (also known as the phrenoesophageal membrane) fix the esophagus to the diaphragm with sufficient laxity to permit the movements of peristalsis. Laxity of this membrane is thought to lead to the development of hiatal hernia.

The reported incidence of hiatal hernia varies depending on the definition used from <10% to more than 20%. Hiatal

hernias may be asymptomatic, may be associated with symptoms of gastroesophageal reflux disease (GERD), or may be associated with acute symptoms of pain and obstruction if the herniated stomach volvulizes.

Hiatal hernias are divided into four types:

Type 1: sliding hiatal hernia; esophagogastric junction and stomach above the diaphragm

Type 2: paraesophageal hernia; esophagogastric junction below the diaphragm, stomach above the diaphragm

Type 3: paraesophageal hernia; esophagogastric junction and stomach above the diaphragm (herniated stomach located alongside the esophagus)

Type 4: paraesophageal hernia; stomach above the diaphragm; also other organs such as the pancreas and bowel contained within the hernia sac

Type 1 hernias account for approximately 90% of hiatal hernias, whereas types 2 to 4 account for approximately 10% of hernias. Type 1 hernias are associated with gastroesophageal reflux, whereas types 2 to 4 are at increased risk for mechanical complications due to volvulus.

Visualization of the longitudinal gastric folds above the diaphragmatic impression or diaphragmatic shadow is diagnostic of a hiatal hernia. The size of the hernia should be approximated by describing which anatomic portions of the stomach (e.g., fundus and body) are located above the diaphragm.

Questions for Further Thought

1. What are the normal contents of the esophageal hiatus?
2. How are sliding hiatal hernias treated?

Reporting Requirements

1. Characterize the hernia as a sliding-type or paraesophageal hernia.
2. Report which segments of the stomach (e.g., fundus and body) are contained within the hernia sac as a way to convey the approximate size of the hernia.

What the Treating Physician Needs to Know

1. Whether the hernia is a sliding type or has a paraesophageal component as paraesophageal hernias are more predisposed to mechanical obstruction due to volvulus.

Answers

1. The esophagus and vagus nerves extend through the esophageal hiatus.
2. Gastroesophageal reflux associated with sliding hiatal hernias is usually initially managed medically. If medical management fails, the sliding hiatal hernia may be surgically repaired via a laparoscopic or open approach. The abnormally enlarged esophageal hiatus may be closed with large sutures ("cruroplasty") or mesh.

REFERENCES

1. Kahrilas PJ, Kim HC, Pandolfino JE. Approaches to the diagnosis and grading of hiatal hernia. Best Pract Res Clin Gastroenterol 2008;22:601-616.
2. Frantzides CT, Madan AK, Carlson MA, Stavropoulos GP. A prospective, randomized trial of laparoscopic polytetrafluoroethylene (PTFE) patch repair vs simple cruroplasty for large hiatal hernia. JAMA Surgery 2002;137:649-652.

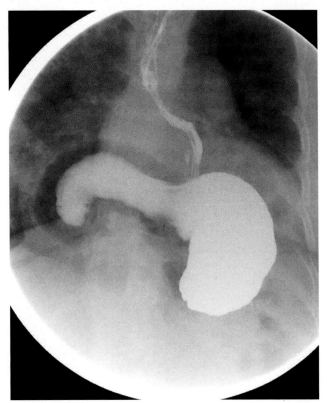

FIGURE 1.4A

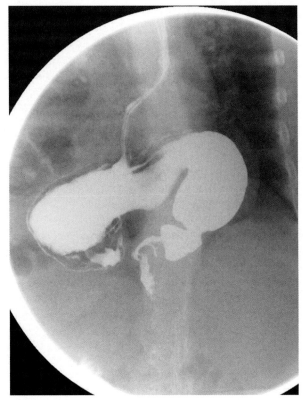

FIGURE 1.4B

FINDINGS Frontal (A) and oblique (B) images from a barium swallow demonstrate the majority of the stomach (including the fundus, body, and antrum) to be located above the diaphragm. The stomach has herniated alongside the esophagus. The esophagogastric junction is located at or just above the diaphragm (B) based on the location of the diaphragmatic shadow. Additionally, the stomach is rotated such that the greater curvature of the stomach is located craniad (organoaxial volvulus). Contrast material empties from the stomach into the duodenum. Note the circumferential lucency around contrast material in the gastric antrum and pylorus indicating wall thickening (A).

DIFFERENTIAL DIAGNOSIS Sliding hiatal hernia, paraesophageal hernia.

DIAGNOSIS Paraesophageal hernia.

DISCUSSION Hiatal hernias are divided into four types:

Type 1: sliding hiatal hernia; esophagogastric junction and stomach above the diaphragm

Type 2: paraesophageal hernia; esophagogastric junction below diaphragm, stomach above the diaphragm

Type 3: paraesophageal hernia; esophagogastric junction and stomach above the diaphragm (herniated stomach located alongside the esophagus)

Type 4: paraesophageal hernia; stomach above the diaphragm; also other organs such as the pancreas and bowel contained within the hernia sac

Paraesophageal hernias are much rarer than sliding-type hiatal hernias and account for approximately 10% of hernias. Type 3 hiatal hernias are the most common paraesophageal hernia. The esophagogastric junction is located above the diaphragm in both type 1 (sliding) and type 3 (paraesophageal) hiatal hernias. Type 3 paraesophageal hernias can be distinguished from type 1 (sliding) hiatal hernias as the herniated stomach is located alongside the esophagus in patients with type 3 hernias.

Distinguishing between a sliding (type 1) and paraesophageal (types 2 to 4) hernia is an important distinction as paraesophageal hernias are more prone to gastric volvulus (as in this case) with resultant mechanical obstruction.

Paraesophageal hernias are more likely to be electively repaired as compared with sliding hiatal hernias given the increased risk of volvulus and mechanical obstruction. Symptomatic paraesophageal hernia (e.g., chest pain, epigastric pain, reflux, and dysphagia) is an indication for elective surgical repair. Acute strangulation, volvulus, and perforation are indications for emergent surgery. Surgical repair includes hernia reduction, diaphragmatic defect closure, and often a fundoplication procedure to help fix the stomach below the diaphragm.

Questions for Further Thought

1. Are paraesophageal hernias more common in younger or older patients?
2. What conditions are thought to predispose to hiatal hernia formation?

Reporting Requirements

1. Report whether the hiatal hernia is a sliding or paraesophageal hernia.
2. Report if there is gastric volvulus.
3. Report if there is gastric outlet obstruction.

What the Treating Physician Needs to Know

1. This patient has a large paraesophageal hernia with organoaxial volvulus.
2. General surgery referral is suggested so patient can be evaluated for repair.

Answers

1. Paraesophageal hernias are more common in elderly individuals.
2. Conditions that weaken the phrenoesophageal ligaments such as increased intra-abdominal pressure because of pregnancy or obesity, repeated episodes of nausea and vomiting, and chronic cough are thought to predispose to hiatal hernia formation.

REFERENCE

1. Bonati H, Neuhauser B, Hinder RA. Para-esophageal hernias. In LeBlanc KA, ed. *Laparoscopic Hernia Surgery: An Operative Guide*. Boca Raton, FL: CRC Press; 2003:201-208.

CLINICAL HISTORY *66-year-old woman with dysphagia.*

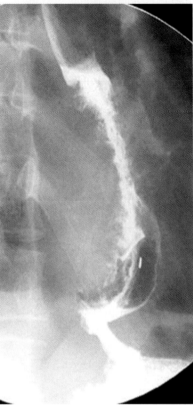

FIGURE 1.5A

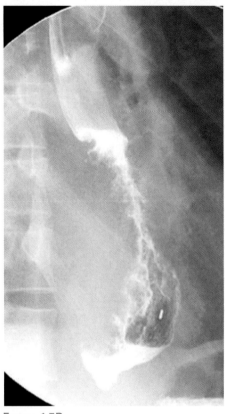

FIGURE 1.5B

FINDINGS Air-contrast barium swallow demonstrates a large, approximately 7-cm segmental area of luminal narrowing and mucosal irregularity involving the distal third of the esophagus (A, B).

DIFFERENTIAL DIAGNOSIS Neoplasm, severe inflammation caused by gastroesophageal reflex disease (GERD).

DIAGNOSIS Neoplasm (adenocarcinoma).

DISCUSSION An estimated 17,990 new cases of esophageal cancer were diagnosed in the United States in 2012, and 15,210 individuals died from the disease. In the United States, adenocarcinoma is the most common esophageal cancer subtype, the distal esophagus is the most common location, and GERD is the most common risk factor. Worldwide, squamous cell carcinoma is the most common subtype, the upper esophagus is the most common location, and alcohol and tobacco use are the major risk factors.

GERD results in chronic esophageal irritation and inflammation which can progress to esophageal metaplasia (also known as Barrett esophagus) and eventually to esophageal cancer. Patients with esophageal cancer often present with dysphagia (difficulty swallowing) and odynophagia (painful swallowing). Raspy cough may also occur if the tumor involves the recurrent laryngeal nerve.

Tumors are generally large by the time they become symptomatic which accounts for the poor prognosis of patients with esophageal cancer. Additionally, the esophagus lacks a serosal layer which normally serves as a barrier to extension of disease elsewhere in the gastrointestinal (GI) tract. Chemoradiation followed by esophagogastrectomy is the usual treatment for distal esophageal cancers. Palliative treatment includes the placement of metallic stents to palliate obstructing lesions.

The hallmark of esophageal malignancy at barium swallow is mucosal irregularity. Mucosal irregularity distinguishes mucosal lesions from submucosal and extrinsic lesions. Compare the mucosal irregularity seen in this case with the predominantly smooth appearance of the mucosa seen with the submucosal masses in other cases in this volume. Esophageal cancers can also appear as plaque-like or polypoid masses.

Question for Further Thought

1. What methods are used to stage esophageal cancer?

Reporting Requirements

1. Describe the location of the abnormality.
2. Recommend EGD and tissue sampling to determine the diagnosis.

What the Treating Physician Needs to Know

1. This patient has a large esophageal mass that is highly suspicious for malignancy.
2. Further evaluation is required with tissue sampling.

3. Whether the mass is obstructing based on the transit of liquid barium and the 12.5-mm compressed barium tablet.

Answer

1. Endoscopic ultrasound (EUS) is used to determine the local extent of disease and sometimes nodal disease. CT and positron emission tomography (PET)/CT are also used to evaluate for nodal disease and to evaluate for metastases (e.g., liver and lung).

REFERENCES

1. www.cancer.gov. Accessed March 5, 2013.
2. Lagergren J, Bergstrom R, Lindgren A, Nyren O. Symptomatic gastroesophageal reflux as a risk factor for esophageal adenocarcinoma. N Engl J Med 1999;340:825-831.
3. Shaheen NJ, Richter JE. Barrett's oesophagus. Lancet 2009;373: 850-861.

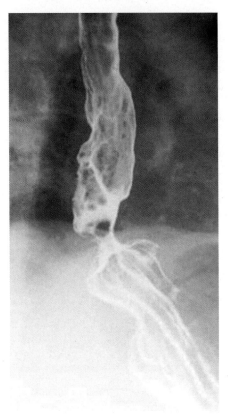

FIGURE 1.6A

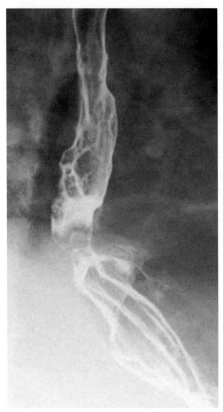

FIGURE 1.6B

FINDINGS Air-contrast barium swallow (A, B) demonstrates an approximately 4-cm segmental plaque-like area of wall thickening and mucosal irregularity involving the distal esophagus.

DIFFERENTIAL DIAGNOSIS Neoplasm, severe inflammation caused by GERD.

DIAGNOSIS Neoplasm (adenocarcinoma).

DISCUSSION The mucosal irregularity seen in this case indicates that this is a mucosal process. This abnormality is compatible with esophageal cancer, and EGD is needed for tissue confirmation. Distal esophageal cancers are most commonly adenocarcinomas. GERD is a major risk factor.

Staging of esophageal cancer often involves endoscopy, CT or PET/CT studies to evaluate local disease extent, nodal stations, and for the presence of distant metastatic disease. Since the esophagus lacks a serosal surface, there is not a significant barrier to prevent esophageal malignancies from directly extending into adjacent structures including the tracheobronchial tree and lung.

The esophagus contains an extensive lymphatic system with bidirectional flow and is unusual in its lymphatic drainage as the esophagus is drained by nodal stations located both above and below the diaphragm. The lymphatics of the upper third of the esophagus, in general, drain craniad with involvement of nodal stations including internal jugular and supraclavicular stations. The lymphatics of the distal third of the esophagus, in general, drain below the diaphragm to involve gastrohepatic ligament and celiac lymph nodes. However, because of bidirectional flow in the extensive esophageal lymphatic plexus distal cancers may result in supraclavicular lymph node disease and vice versa.

Location of hematogeneous metastases in decreasing order of frequency are as follows: liver, lungs, bones, adrenal glands, kidneys, and brain.

Questions for Further Thought

1. Describe the different morphologies of esophageal cancer seen at barium swallow.
2. What modality is recommended to determine the depth of tumor invasion?

Reporting Requirements

1. Describe the location of the abnormality.
2. Recommend EGD and tissue sampling to determine the diagnosis.

What the Treating Physician Needs to Know

1. This patient has a large esophageal mass that is highly suspicious for malignancy.
2. Further evaluation is required with tissue sampling.

Answers

1. Esophageal cancers may appear as areas of mucosal irregularity, plaque-like lesions, or polypoid lesions.

2. EUS is used to determine the depth of tumor invasion and is often used to evaluate for disease in regional lymph nodes.

REFERENCES

1. www.cancer.gov. Accessed March 5, 2013.
2. Levine MS, Rubesin SE. Diseases of the esophagus: diagnosis with esophagography. Radiology 2005;237:414-427.
3. Sharma A, Fidias P, Hayman LA, Loomis SL, Taber KH, Aquino SL. Patterns of lymphadenopathy in thoracic malignancies. Radiographics 2004;24:419-434.

CLINICAL HISTORY *68-year-old man with history of GERD.*

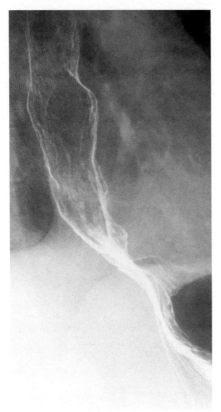

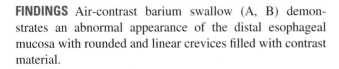

FIGURE 1.7A

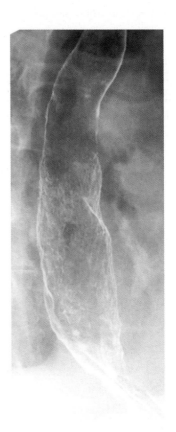

FIGURE 1.7B

FINDINGS Air-contrast barium swallow (A, B) demonstrates an abnormal appearance of the distal esophageal mucosa with rounded and linear crevices filled with contrast material.

DIFFERENTIAL DIAGNOSIS Barrett esophagus, esophageal adenocarcinoma.

DIAGNOSIS Barrett esophagus.

DISCUSSION At fluoroscopy, a reticular mucosal pattern with barium filling thin grooves or crevices is a highly specific but insensitive sign of Barrett esophagus. Barrett esophagus is defined as metaplasia with columnar epithelium replacing the usual esophageal squamous epithelium. The squamocolumnar junction is displaced proximally in patients with Barrett esophagus. Diagnosis is made based on mucosal biopsies at EGD.

Barrett esophagus is considered to be a premalignant condition. This abnormality is found in approximately 10% to 15% of adults with GERD who undergo endoscopy. Barrett esophagus is found in the majority of patients with esophageal and gastroesophageal cancers in the United States.

Most major GI societies recommend endoscopic surveillance of patients with Barrett esophagus at 1- to 3-year intervals to include detailed inspection of the esophageal mucosa and systematic biopsies. Treatment of Barrett esophagus includes medical management of GERD and antireflux surgery (e.g., hiatal hernia reduction and Nissen fundoplication) for patients who do not respond to medical management.

Barrett esophagus is named after Norman Barrett (1903 to 1979), a thoracic surgeon who described the condition in 1950.

Questions for Further Thought

1. What percentage of patients with reflux esophagitis develop Barrett esophagus?
2. What percentage of patients with Barrett esophagus develop esophageal cancer?

Reporting Requirements

1. Describe the location and approximate length of disease.
2. Recommend that EGD and possibly tissue sampling be performed.

What the Treating Physician Needs to Know

1. EGD with tissue sampling is needed to confirm the diagnosis of Barrett esophagus.

Answers

1. Approximately 10% of patients with reflux esophagitis will develop Barrett esophagus.

2. Roughly 0.5% of patients with Barrett esophagus per year develop esophageal adenocarcinoma.

REFERENCES

1. Levine MS, Rubesin SE. Diseases of the esophagus: diagnosis with esophagography. Radiology 2005;237:414-427.
2. Sharma P. Barrett's esophagus. N Engl J Med 2009;361: 2548-2556.

CLINICAL HISTORY *57-year-old man with no known past medical history presents with chest pain.*

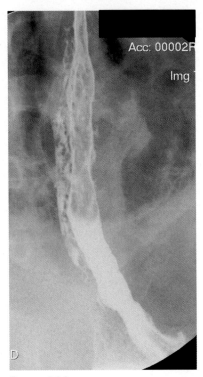

FIGURE 1.8A

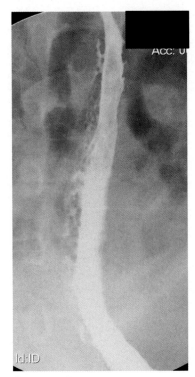

FIGURE 1.8B

FINDINGS Air-contrast barium swallow demonstrates extensive mucosal irregularity of the mid- and distal esophagus with extensive ulcerations (A, B).

DIFFERENTIAL DIAGNOSIS *Candida* esophagitis, reflux esophagitis, Crohn esophagitis.

DIAGNOSIS *Candida* esophagitis.

DISCUSSION *Candida albicans* is the most common etiology of infectious esophagitis. The earliest manifestation of *Candida* esophagitis is esophageal dysmotility. The esophageal mucosa may appear normal at barium swallow early in the disease. As esophageal candidiasis worsens in severity, mucosal plaques may be visible followed by erosions and ulcerations. The above image is from a patient with very advanced disease. Crohn esophagitis could have a similar appearance, and EGD with biopsy was required to confirm the diagnosis.

Patients who develop candidiasis usually have a predisposing condition including immunosuppression (e.g., due to human immunodeficiency virus [HIV], steroids, chemotherapy, or transplant patients) or patients who have delayed esophageal emptying (e.g., due to esophageal strictures, scleroderma, or achalasia).

Treatment of esophageal candidiasis is with fluconazole or itraconazole.

Question for Further Thought

1. What would be the next step to establish the diagnosis?

Reporting Requirements

1. Describe the location of the mucosal abnormality.
2. Suggest EGD for further evaluation and possible tissue sampling.

What the Treating Physician Needs to Know

1. The imaging findings, though markedly abnormal, are nonspecific and EGD is needed for definitive diagnosis.

Answer

1. Endoscopy with possible tissue sampling would be the next step to establish the diagnosis.

REFERENCES

1. Roberts L, Gibbons R, Gibbons G, et al. Adult esophageal candidiasis: a radiographic spectrum. Radiographics 1987;7: 289-307.
2. Pappas PG, Rex JH, Sobel JD, et al. Guidelines for treatment of candidiasis. Clin Infect Dis 2004;38:161-189.

CASE 1.9

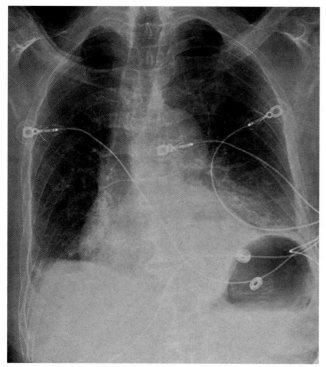

FIGURE 1.9A

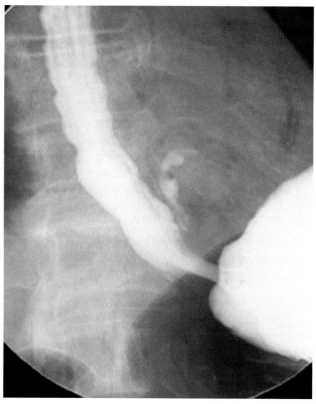

FIGURE 1.9B

FINDINGS Initial chest radiograph (A) obtained in the emergency department demonstrates a retrocardiac air–fluid level. Differential diagnosis for this finding includes air–fluid level in a hiatal hernia versus in the pleural space due to esophageal rupture. A chest CT was performed (not shown) which demonstrated pneumomediastinum along with fluid and air in the left pleural space. Given CT findings and clinical history, there was a high level of concern for esophageal rupture. The patient underwent a swallow study which showed a somewhat linear collection of contrast material arising from and extending away from the left side of the distal esophagus (B).

DIFFERENTIAL DIAGNOSIS Boerhaave syndrome, Mallory-Weiss tear.

DIAGNOSIS Boerhaave syndrome.

DISCUSSION Boerhaave syndrome is defined as rupture of the esophageal wall due to vomiting. A proposed mechanism is failure of normal relaxation of the cricopharyngeus muscle during vomiting leading to increased intraesophageal pressure and rupture. The resultant esophageal tear is usually oriented longitudinally, 1 to 4 cm in length, and located in the left lateral wall of the distal esophagus just proximal to the esophagogastric junction.

At plain film, pneumomediastinum, left pleural fluid, and subcutaneous emphysema may be seen. These same findings are also visible at chest CT. In the appropriate clinical setting, these findings are highly suggestive of Boerhaave syndrome. Esophagography is the definitive imaging test. Treatment includes surgical repair and antibiotic therapy. Untreated, mortality is assumed to be 100%. With treatment, mortality rates are reduced to <20%.

A Mallory-Weiss tear differs from Boerhaave syndrome as a Mallory-Weiss tear only involves the esophageal mucosa. In other words, with a Mallory-Weiss tear no esophageal leak will be seen at fluoroscopy. Mallory-Weiss tears are difficult to diagnose with esophagography. Like the esophageal perforations associated with Boerhaave syndrome, Mallory-Weiss tears usually involve the distal esophagus.

Boerhaave syndrome is named after physician Hermann Boerhaave (1668 to 1738) based on his detailed description of the condition in a 1724 manuscript.

Questions for Further Thought

1. What contrast agent(s) should be used to evaluate for a possible esophageal rupture?
2. What contrast agent(s) should be used to evaluate for possible aspiration?

Reporting Requirements

1. Immediately contact the clinical team regarding the chest radiograph to convey concern regarding possible air in the pleural space indicating an esophageal perforation. Chest CT is a reasonable recommendation following the chest radiograph to confirm that the retrocardiac air is in the pleural space rather than a hiatal hernia.
2. Immediately contact the clinical team following the esophagram to inform them of the esophageal rupture.

What the Treating Physician Needs to Know

1. This patient has a perforated esophagus.
2. Cardiothoracic surgery (or thoracic surgery) consultation is needed.

Answers

1. Water-soluble contrast material should be used initially, after confirming that the patient is not allergic to iodine. Rationale for beginning with water-soluble contrast material is that if barium leaks into the mediastinum it will not be resorbed and may result in mediastinitis. By comparison, water-soluble contrast material will be resorbed if it leaks into the mediastinum. The goal is to first exclude a large leak with water-soluble contrast material. If the initial water-soluble contrast material images are negative for leak (as in this case, images not shown), the patient should drink thin barium. Rationale is that barium (as in this case) sometimes demonstrates leaks that are not seen with water-soluble contrast material. One theory for why barium is more effective than water-soluble contrast material for demonstrating leaks is that patients will take larger gulps of barium as it is less foul-tasting than water-soluble contrast material. These larger gulps of barium distend the esophagus more than small sips of water-soluble contrast material and may demonstrate a leak not visible with water-soluble contrast material. Additionally, barium is denser than water-soluble contrast material and is therefore better seen at fluoroscopy.

2. If concern is for aspiration, the patient should consume small sips of thin barium. Rationale is that aspiration of water-soluble contrast material can result in a severe pneumonitis or pulmonary edema, whereas barium is more inert. If the patient is observed to aspirate barium, the patient should be instructed to cough up as much as possible.

REFERENCES

1. Kanne JP, Rohrmann CA Jr, Lichtenstein JE. Eponyms in radiology of the digestive tract: historical perspectives and imaging appearances. Part 1. pharynx, esophagus, stomach and intestine. Radiographics 2006;26:129-142.
2. Teh E, Edwards J, Duffy J, Beggs D. Boerhaave's syndrome: a review of management and outcome. Interact CardioVasc Thorac Surg 2007;6:640-643.

CASE 1.10

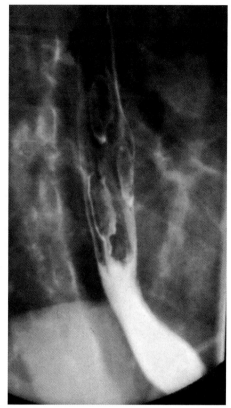

Figure 1.10

FINDINGS Air-contrast barium swallow demonstrates three large, approximately 3-cm ulcers in the mid-esophagus.

DIFFERENTIAL DIAGNOSIS HIV ulcer, cytomegalovirus (CMV) ulcer, herpes simplex virus (HSV) ulcer, pill-induced ulcer.

DIAGNOSIS CMV ulcer.

DISCUSSION Large ulcers are defined as ulcers greater than 1 cm. The differential diagnosis of large ulcers in an HIV-positive patient includes CMV and HIV infection. HSV may also present as ulcers at fluoroscopy, but HSV ulcers are typically less than 1 cm in size. Pill-induced ulcers are also typically small in size.

At fluoroscopy, CMV disease of the esophagus may manifest as large ulcers or a more diffuse esophagitis. In the HIV population, CMV infections usually occur in patients with advanced immunosuppression and CD4 counts <50. Since the introduction of highly active antiretroviral therapy (HAART), CMV end-organ infection has become quite rare with 6 cases per 100 person-years reported in recent series. Of these acquired immunodeficiency syndrome (AIDS) patients who experience end-organ CMV disease, approximately 5% to 10% will develop CMV esophagitis. Such patients typically present with fever, odynophagia, nausea, and chest pain.

As treatment of CMV esophagitis normally requires peripherally inserted central catheter line placement and a 21- to 28-day course of intravenous foscarnet or ganciclovir, endoscopy with tissue sampling is usually performed to distinguish between a CMV ulcer and an HIV ulcer.

Question for Further Thought

1. What would be the next step to confirm the diagnosis?

Reporting Requirement

1. Describe the size and location of ulcers.

What the Treating Physician Needs to Know

1. That a large ulcer in an HIV-positive patient may be caused by HIV disease or CMV.

Answer

1. Endoscopy and biopsy would be the steps to establish a diagnosis.

REFERENCES

1. Rubesin SE, Levine MS. Differential diagnosis of esophageal disease on esophagography. Appl Radiol 2001;10:11-21.
2. Balthazar EJ, Megibow AJ, Hulnick DH. Cytomegalovirus esophagitis and gastritis in AIDS. Am J Roentgenol 1985;144: 1201-1204.
3. Kaplan JE, Benson C, Holmes KK, Brooks JT, Pau A, Masur H. Guidelines for prevention and treatment of opportunistic infections in HIV-infected adults and adolescents. Morb Mortal Wkly Rep 2009;58:1-198.

CLINICAL HISTORY *35-year-old woman with dysphagia.*

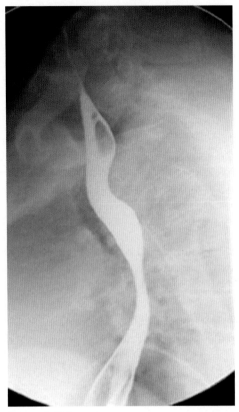

FIGURE 1.11A

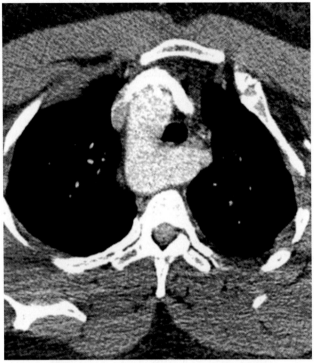

FIGURE 1.11C

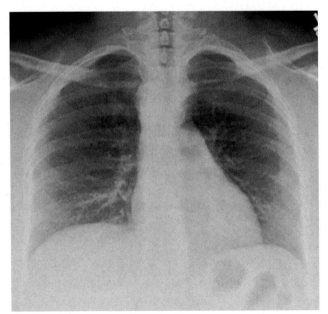

FIGURE 1.11B

FINDINGS Lateral image from a barium swallow (A) demonstrates a smooth impression on the posterior aspect of the proximal esophagus. Frontal chest radiograph (B) demonstrates mass effect along the right side of the trachea. Contrast-enhanced CT image (C) demonstrates a diverticulum of Kommerell and an aberrant left subclavian artery arising from a right-sided aortic arch. This vessel passes posterior to the trachea and esophagus.

DIFFERENTIAL DIAGNOSIS BASED ON BARIUM SWALLOW Submucosal mass, extrinsic compression.

DIAGNOSIS Extrinsic compression on esophagus due to aberrant left subclavian artery, also right-sided aortic arch.

DISCUSSION The above area of mass effect seen at barium swallow has a "marble under the rug" appearance indicating that it is a submucosal mass or extrinsic process. The smoothness of the mucosa also excludes a mucosally based process.

The key to making this diagnosis is an awareness of the possibility of an aberrant subclavian artery running behind the esophagus. Chest CT would be the next best step in this case to confirm and better delineate the patient's vascular anatomy. Mistakenly recommending EGD with biopsy in this case could result in catastrophic bleeding.

The two most common vascular rings reported in adults are double aortic arch and right-sided aortic arch with aberrant left subclavian artery. Patients with these conditions may present with symptoms related to the respiratory track (e.g., dyspnea on exertion or stridor) or with dysphagia. Some patients may be asymptomatic.

Questions for Further Thought

1. What is dysphagia lusoria?
2. What would be treatment options for the above-described patient?

Reporting Requirements

1. Inform the ordering clinician of the abnormal study.
2. Recommend chest CT to evaluate for vascular ring.

What the Treating Physician Needs to Know

1. The extrinsic esophageal mass could be a vascular structure, and therefore EGD with biopsy should *not* be performed as the next step in diagnosis.

2. This patient may be asymptomatic or experience symptoms related to the respiratory or GI tracts.

Answers

1. The term "dysphagia lusoria" originates from the Latin word "lusus naturae," which means "freak of nature," and is most commonly defined as compression of the esophagus due to an aberrant right subclavian artery running behind the esophagus.
2. If a vascular ring is asymptomatic, no treatment is warranted. The above patient reported symptoms of dysphagia and shortness of breath. At barium swallow, there was no impairment to the transit of liquid barium or the barium tablet. However, because of her reported symptoms and concern for eventual aneurysm rupture, the patient underwent surgical repair which included repairing the diverticulum of Kommerell with an aortic graft and then anastomosing the left subclavian artery to the aortic graft.

REFERENCES

1. Kent PD, Poterucha TH. Aberrant right subclavian artery and dysphagia lusoria. N Engl J Med 2002;346:1637.
2. Grathwohl KW, Afifi AY, Dillard TA, Olson JP, Heric BR. Vascular rings of the thoracic aorta in adults. Am Surg 1999;65: 1077-1083.

CLINICAL HISTORY *67-year-old woman with dysphagia and experiencing episodes of regurgitation of a large sausage-like mass which she could not expel.*

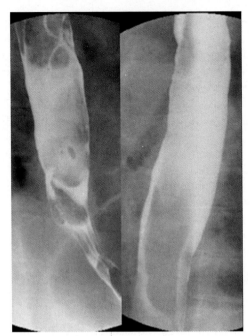

FIGURE 1.12A

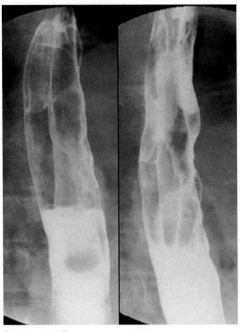

FIGURE 1.12B

FINDINGS Air-contrast barium swallow study demonstrates multiple smooth, expansile, sausage-shaped masses (A, B). Contrast material coats all sides of the masses, and the masses were mobile during real-time imaging.

DIFFERENTIAL DIAGNOSIS Fibrovascular polyps, leiomyomas.

DIAGNOSIS Fibrovascular polyps.

DISCUSSION Fibrovascular polyps are rare benign tumors. These tumors usually arise near the level of the crico-pharyngeus muscle and gradually elongate over a period of years as they are dragged inferiorly due to esophageal peristalsis.

Patients sometimes present with weight loss and retrosternal pain. Polyp ulceration can result in bleeding. The patient may experience regurgitation of a lobulated mass with a broad stalk. In some cases, airway obstruction and asphyxia have been reported.

At fluoroscopy, fibrovascular polyps appear as intraluminal filling defects. An intraluminal location is suggested by the presence of contrast material coating all sides of the mass in multiple projections. Also, as fibrovascular polyps are usually tethered by a stalk, they often appear mobile at barium swallow. By comparison, leiomyomas typically do not appear polypoid but more often have a "marble under the rug" appearance.

Question for Further Thought

1. What are treatment options for fibrovascular polyps?

Reporting Requirements

1. Describe the size and location of the lesions.
2. Attempt to characterize the lesions as intraluminal in location which favors a diagnosis of fibrovascular polyps.

What the Treating Physician Needs to Know

1. This patient has intraluminal esophageal masses that are most likely fibrovascular polyps.
2. Surgical resection likely will be necessary to alleviate patient symptoms.

Answer

1. Depending on the size of the polyp, it may be amenable to endoscopic excision. Alternatively, a thoracotomy may be required to remove larger polyps.

REFERENCES

1. Levine MS, Rubesin SE. Diseases of the esophagus: diagnosis with esophagography. Radiology 2005;237:414-427.
2. Morin FD, Bret PM, Gret P, Palayew MJ. General case of the day: Fibrovascular polyp of the esophagus. Radiographics 1992;12:845-847.
3. Jang GC, Clouse ME, Fleischner FG. Fibrovascular polyps–a benign intraluminal tumor of the esophagus. Radiology 1969;92:1196-1200.

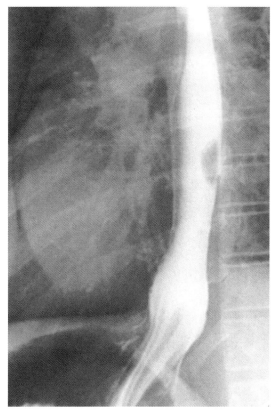

FIGURE 1.13A

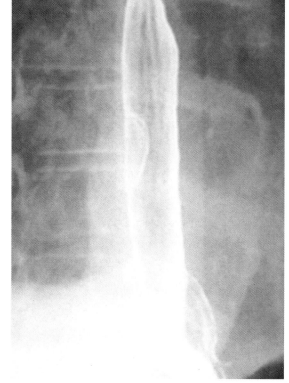

FIGURE 1.13B

FINDINGS Single-contrast image (A) demonstrates a 2-cm contour abnormality in the middle to lower third of the esophagus. The contour abnormality has the appearance of a "marble under a rug" with respect to the esophageal lumen. The esophageal mucosa is smooth, best seen in the air-contrast image (B).

DIFFERENTIAL DIAGNOSIS Submucosal mass (-omas: lipoma, leiomyoma, neuroma, fibroma, neurofibroma), extrinsic compression (lymph node, vascular structure, duplication cyst).

DIAGNOSIS Submucosal mass (granular cell tumor).

DISCUSSION The smooth mucosa and "marble under a rug" appearance make a mucosal abnormality extremely unlikely. A submucosal mass rather than an area of extrinsic compression can be favored by noting the normal outer contour of the esophagus at this level. By comparison, areas of extrinsic compression often distort the outer esophageal contour.

As a radiologist, you have done your job by identifying the abnormality as a submucosal mass for which CT

(to evaluate for a fat containing lipoma) or EUS with possible tissue sampling could be performed as the next step to establish the diagnosis.

Granular cell tumors of the esophagus are rare tumors and are thought to be of neurogenic origin. Diagnosis is made based on endoscopic biopsy. Granular cell tumors have been reported in a variety of locations, including the skin, larynx, breast, and vulva. The "granularity" of these tumors is caused by accumulation of lysosomes in the cytoplasm.

When located in the esophagus, granular cell tumors most frequently occur in the distal esophagus and are usually small at the time of detection with 75% <1 cm in size in one series. In many patients with small granular cell tumors, these tumors are thought to be an incidental finding at the time of endoscopy rather than the actual cause of the patient's dysphagia. Granular cell tumors are not thought to produce dysphagia until they reach at least 1 cm in size.

A literature search for granular cell tumors of the esophagus reveals a smattering of case reports and case series. Given the relative rarity of this tumor, the best treatment strategy is yet to be defined. In general, once the diagnosis of a granular cell tumor is made with endoscopic biopsy, periodic surveillance with endoscopy or fluoroscopy is thought to be adequate to assess for size stability. The optimal surveillance frequency is yet to be defined. If tumor removal is desired, endoscopic and surgical removal are options.

Question for Further Thought

1. What is the management of esophageal granular cell tumors?

Reporting Requirements

1. Describe the location of the abnormality.
2. Recommend EUS with possible tissue sampling or cross-sectional imaging (to evaluate for lipoma) for further evaluation.

What the Treating Physician Needs to Know

1. The patient has a submucosal esophageal mass.

2. Whether the mass is obstructing based on transit of liquid barium and the 12.5-mm compressed barium tablet past the level of the mass.

Answer

1. Esophageal granular cell tumors are such rare tumors that appropriate management is somewhat controversial. These benign tumors are thought to have no malignant potential. Therefore, a conservative approach with periodic (often yearly) surveillance to confirm size stability is suggested in patients with small (<1 cm), asymptomatic tumors.

REFERENCES

1. Goldblum JR, Rice TW, Zuccaro G, Richter JE. Granular cell tumors of the esophagus: a clinical and pathologic study of 13 cases. Ann Thorac Surg 1996;62:860-865.
2. Voskull JH, van Dijk MM, Wagenaar SS, van Vilet AC, Timmer R, van Hees PA. Occurrence of esophageal granular cell tumors in The Netherlands between 1998 and 1994. Dig Dis Sci 2001;46:1610-1614.

CLINICAL HISTORY *54-year-old man with dysphagia.*

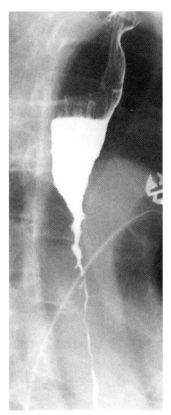

FIGURE 1.14A

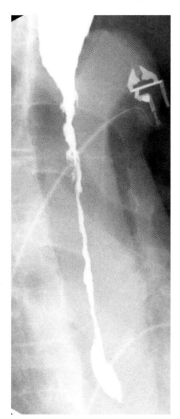

FIGURE 1.14B

FINDINGS Fluoroscopic images from a single-contrast barium swallow (A, B) demonstrate a long-segment fixed narrowing of the mid- and distal esophagus.

DIFFERENTIAL DIAGNOSIS Esophageal stricture, esophageal cancer.

DIAGNOSIS Long-segment esophageal stricture.

DISCUSSION The smooth margins of the more distal area of fixed narrowing favor a benign stricture rather than malignancy. EGD should be recommended to distinguish a benign from a malignant stricture in most cases.

Esophageal strictures result from long-standing esophageal inflammation leading to fibrosis. Strictures can be classified based on their location as well as whether they are long-segment or short-segment strictures. Historically, GERD was the etiology of the majority of esophageal strictures in the United States and could produce long-segment or short-segment strictures. Due to improved medical management options for GERD, reflux-induced strictures have declined in frequency.

Other potential etiologies of long-segment strictures include caustic ingestion and radiation. Patients with long-standing indwelling nasogastric tubes can also develop long-segment distal esophageal strictures due to the tube preventing closure of the lower esophageal sphincter with resultant reflux of acidic gastric contents into the distal esophagus. Scleroderma patients also may develop a nonfunctioning lower esophageal sphincter due to smooth muscle atrophy with resultant spontaneous gastroesophageal reflux, inflammation, and eventual stricture formation.

Whether or not a 12.5-mm compressed barium tablet passes through a stricture can be used to assess the esophageal luminal diameter in the area of the stricture.

Questions for Further Thought

1. Name three etiologies of short-segment esophageal strictures.
2. What is the usual treatment for a benign esophageal stricture?

Reporting Requirements

1. Describe the length and location of the stricture.

2. Based on stricture length and location, suggest the potential causative etiologies.
3. Recommend EGD to exclude malignancy in most cases.

What the Treating Physician Needs to Know

1. Whether the stricture appears benign or malignant. If uncertain, EGD should be recommended for further evaluation.

Answers

1. Reflux esophagitis, medication-induced, and esophageal cancer are etiologies of short-segment strictures.

2. First-line treatment of a benign esophageal stricture is endoscopic dilatation using either a bougie (a cylindrical instrument used for dilatation) or a balloon. Stents may be placed in patients whose strictures are refractory to dilatation.

REFERENCES

1. Luedtke P, Levine MS, Rubesin SE, Weinstein DS, Laufer I. Radiologic diagnosis of benign esophageal strictures: a pattern approach. Radiographics 2003;23:897-909.
2. Baron TH. Management of benign esophageal strictures. Gastroenterol Hepatol 2011;7:46-49.

CLINICAL HISTORY *56-year-old man with dysphagia.*

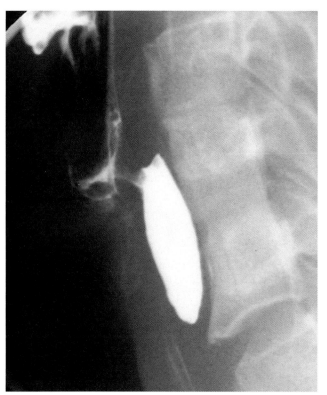

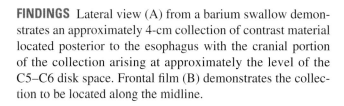

FIGURE 1.15A

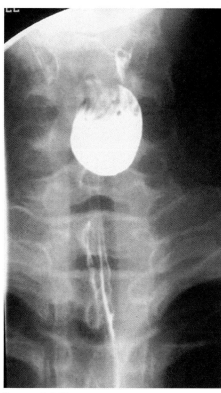

FIGURE 1.15B

FINDINGS Lateral view (A) from a barium swallow demonstrates an approximately 4-cm collection of contrast material located posterior to the esophagus with the cranial portion of the collection arising at approximately the level of the C5–C6 disk space. Frontal film (B) demonstrates the collection to be located along the midline.

DIFFERENTIAL DIAGNOSIS Zenker diverticulum, perforation.

DIAGNOSIS Zenker diverticulum.

DISCUSSION Zenker diverticula originate just proximal to the cricopharyngeus muscle. These diverticula occur when a portion of the esophageal wall herniates through the space between the inferior pharyngeal constrictor and the cricopharyngeus muscle. The etiology of Zenker diverticula is unclear although failure of normal relaxation of the cricopharyngeus muscle has been postulated. With smaller diverticula, the hypopharynx and esophagus remain in line. However, as these diverticula enlarge, they push the lumen of the esophagus anteriorly resulting in dysphagia. Pooling of contrast material in a Zenker diverticulum can be a source of aspiration.

A Zenker diverticulum can be distinguished from a perforation as contrast material will readily fill and empty from a diverticulum, whereas contrast material usually will continue to accumulate at a site of perforation. Diverticula usually demonstrate a smooth, rounded morphology, whereas sites of perforation are more irregular in shape.

Zenker diverticula are named after pathologist Friedrich Alber von Zenker (1825 to 1898).

Questions for Further Thought

1. What are common symptoms in patients with Zenker diverticula?
2. What are current treatment options for Zenker diverticula?

Reporting Requirements

1. Report the approximate size of the diverticulum.
2. Report if the diverticulum narrows the esophageal lumen.

What the Treating Physician Needs to Know

1. Zenker diverticula can be asymptomatic if small but are usually symptomatic when large.

Answers

1. Dysphagia, regurgitation of undigested food hours after eating, halitosis, and aspiration are relatively common complications of Zenker diverticula. Bleeding, fistula

formation, and development of squamous cell carcinomas in the diverticulum are less common complications.

2. Small (<2 cm) diverticula in asymptomatic patients often are not treated. Surgical options for larger, symptomatic diverticula include diverticulectomy.

REFERENCE

1. Grant PD, Morgan DE, Scholz FJ, Canon CL. Pharyngeal dysphagia: what the radiologist needs to know. Curr Probl Diagn Radiol 2009;38:17-32.

CLINICAL HISTORY *38-year-old man with HIV disease and dysphagia.*

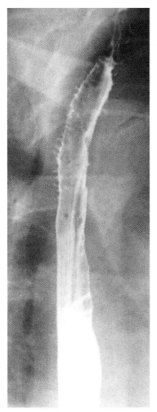

FIGURE 1.16A

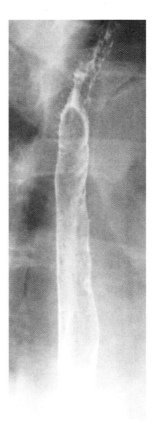

FIGURE 1.16B

FINDINGS Air-contrast barium swallow (A, B) demonstrates numerous relatively parallel, linear outpouchings of contrast material arising from the esophageal lumen. These outpouchings are oriented perpendicular to the long axis of the esophagus.

DIFFERENTIAL DIAGNOSIS Intramural pseudodiverticulosis.

DIAGNOSIS Intramural pseudodiverticulosis.

DISCUSSION Esophageal intramural pseudodiverticulosis is a rare condition that is present in fewer than 1% of swallow studies. The pathogenesis of pseudodiverticulosis is unknown. At histology, dilated submucosal glands and excretory ducts are visible. Pseudodiverticula are thought to reflect contrast material within these dilated excretory ducts.

At barium swallow, pseudodiverticulosis is characterized by numerous small contrast-filled outpouchings located parallel to each other but perpendicular to the esophageal lumen. The outpouchings sometimes appear flask-shaped, though not in the above case. These outpouchings may involve the esophagus diffusely or segmentally, and a relatively equal distribution of segmental disease along the proximal, mid-, and distal esophagus has been described.

Intramural pseudodiverticulosis has been described in association with a number of conditions, including strictures, reflux esophagitis, esophageal candidiasis, acid injury, and esophageal cancer. Patients with esophageal pseudodiverticulosis often present with dysphagia or chest pain though symptoms are usually attributed to conditions such as reflux that accompany pseudodiverticulosis rather than the outpouchings themselves.

Questions for Further Thought

1. What is the treatment of esophageal intramural pseudodiverticulosis?
2. Are these pseudodiverticula expected to resolve with treatment?

Reporting Requirements

1. Report the location of esophageal pseudodiverticulosis.
2. Suggest that EGD may be necessary to determine the underlying etiology.

What the Treating Physician Needs to Know

1. Esophageal intramural pseudodiverticulosis is associated with a variety of usually benign conditions.
2. EGD may be necessary to diagnose the underlying condition.

Answers

1. Treatment is not directed specifically at the pseudodiverticula but rather at the associated condition such as reflux esophagitis or candidiasis.

2. Pseudodiverticula usually resolve with successful treatment of the accompanying condition.

REFERENCES

1. Levine MS, Moolten DN, Herlinger H, Laufer I. Esophageal intramural pseudodiverticulosis: a reevaluation. Am J Roentgenol 1986;147:1165-1170.
2. Levine MS, Rubesin SE. Diseases of the esophagus: diagnosis with esophagography. Radiology 2005;237:414-427.
3. Chon YE, Hwang S, Jung KS, et al. A case of esophageal intramural pseudodiverticulosis. Gut Liver 2011;5:93-95.

CASE 1.17

CLINICAL HISTORY *48-year-old man with HIV disease, dysphagia, and chest pain.*

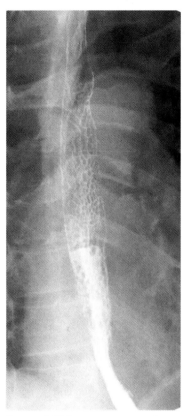

FIGURE 1.17A

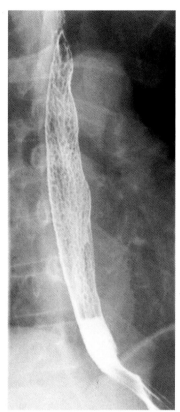

FIGURE 1.17B

FINDINGS Air-contrast barium swallow demonstrates a diffusely abnormal appearance of the esophageal mucosa. Numerous plaque-like areas are seen with thin linear areas of contrast material in between these plaque-like areas (A, B).

DIFFERENTIAL DIAGNOSIS Candidiasis, glycogenic acanthosis, reflux esophagitis, superficial esophageal malignancy.

DIAGNOSIS Candidiasis.

DISCUSSION Esophageal candidiasis is common in HIV-positive patients and is most commonly seen when the CD4 count is <200. *C. albicans* is the most common causative species and usually responds to fluconazole or itraconazole. Esophageal candidiasis is sometimes asymptomatic but usually results in odynophagia.

At physical examination, oropharyngeal candidiasis (also known as "thrush") appears as white plaques that can be scraped off. Esophageal candidiasis has a similar appearance at EGD. At fluoroscopy, esophageal candidiasis may initially manifest as esophageal dysmotility or as raised plaque-like areas as in this case. With more severe disease, the esophagus may develop a "shaggy" appearance. Other conditions that lead to immunocompromise (e.g., diabetes) or stasis (e.g., achalasia or obstructing masses) also can result in candidiasis.

Glycogenic acanthosis may also result in raised plaque-like areas. Glycogenic acanthosis is a benign and usually asymptomatic condition characterized by intracellular glycogen accumulation. This condition most commonly affects elderly patients. Reflux esophagitis may also result in nodular or plaque-like raised areas, most commonly located in the distal esophagus. Superficial esophageal cancer can also appear as raised, plaque-like areas.

Questions for Further Thought

1. Is endoscopy required to confirm esophageal candidiasis prior to treatment in AIDS patients with oral thrush?
2. How can plaques be distinguished from ulcers at fluoroscopy?

Reporting Requirements

1. Describe the presence of diffuse plaque-like areas throughout the esophagus.
2. Suggest that clinical correlation be made for possible candidiasis.

What the Treating Physician Needs to Know

1. In an HIV-positive patient with oral thrush, the above appearance can be assumed to be due to esophageal candidiasis.

2. In other clinical scenarios, EGD with tissue sampling may be necessary to establish a diagnosis prior to treatment.

Answers

1. No. If oral thrush is present and esophageal symptoms are reported, esophageal candidiasis is assumed. Endoscopy is usually unnecessary and is only performed if such patients do not respond to treatment for candidiasis.

2. Plaques are raised areas. At esophagography, contrast material outlines the edges of plaques. On the other hand, ulcers are depressed areas. At esophagography, contrast material is present centrally within an ulcer.

REFERENCES

1. Rubesin SE, Levine MS. Differential diagnosis of esophageal disease on esophagography. Appl Radiol 2001;30:11-21.

2. Bianchi Porro G, Parente F, Cermuschi M. The diagnosis of esophageal candidiasis in patients with acquired immune deficiency syndrome: is endoscopy always necessary? Am J Gastroenterol 1989;84:143-146.

3. Kaplan JE, Benson C, Holmes KK, Brooks JT, Pau A, Masur H. Guidelines for prevention and treatment of opportunistic infections in HIV-infected adults and adolescents. Morb Mortal Wkly Rep 2009;58:1-198.

CLINICAL HISTORY *80-year-old man with abdominal pain.*

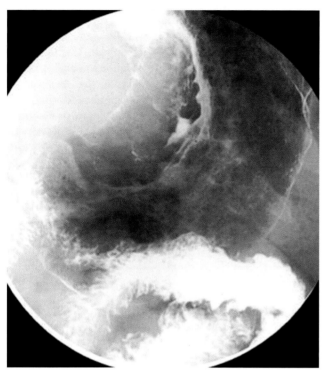

FIGURE 1.18A

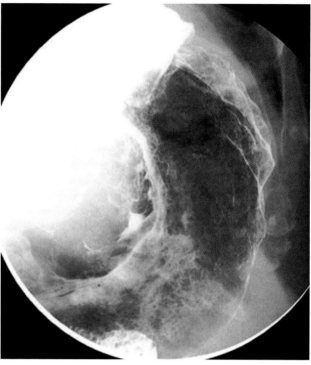

FIGURE 1.18B

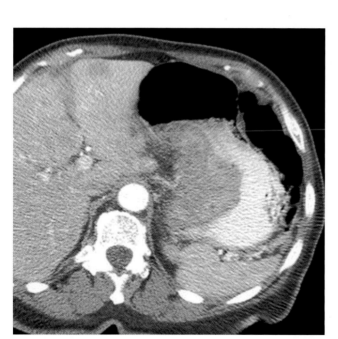

FIGURE 1.18C

FINDINGS Fluoroscopic images (A, B) from an upper GI evaluation demonstrate a 9-cm mass along the lesser curvature of the stomach with mucosal irregularity. CT image (C) with intravenous and oral contrast material demonstrates a 6 cm × 9 cm mass along the lesser curvature of the stomach, invasion of perigastric fat, and liver metastases.

DIFFERENTIAL DIAGNOSIS Gastric adenocarcinoma, lymphoma.

DIAGNOSIS Gastric adenocarcinoma.

DISCUSSION Mucosal irregularity indicates that the mass involves the mucosa. The differential diagnosis is therefore narrowed to adenocarcinoma and lymphoma. The vast majority of gastric malignancies are adenocarcinomas.

Gastric cancer is the third most common GI malignancy in the United States following colorectal cancer and pancreatic cancer. Gastric cancers usually produce no symptoms when small and potentially curable. As gastric malignancies enlarge, patients may experience vague abdominal pain, anorexia, and weight loss. Unfortunately most patients with gastric cancer in the United States present with relatively late stage disease. Five-year survival is 10% to 30% even in patients who undergo surgery which is intended to be curative.

Nodal stations that can be involved with gastric cancer include perigastric nodes (along the lesser and greater curvature, fundus, and pylorus), intermediate nodes (along the left gastric, common hepatic, and celiac arteries), and distant lymph nodes (in the splenic hilum, retropancreatic, mesenteric root, and para-aortic regions). The liver is the most common site of extranodal, distant metastatic disease.

Questions for Further Thought

1. What are Krukenberg tumors?
2. What is Virchow's node?
3. What is a Sister Mary Joseph nodule?

Reporting Requirements

1. Report the size and location of the abnormality.
2. Notify the ordering physician that this patient has an abnormality which is highly suspicious for a gastric malignancy, statistically most likely an adenocarcinoma.

What the Treating Physician Needs to Know

1. This patient most likely has a gastric cancer.
2. Tissue sampling should be performed.

Answers

1. Krukenberg tumors are metastases that involve the ovaries. Gastric adenocarcinomas are the most common source of Krukenberg tumors along with other GI malignancies and breast cancer. Friedrich Krukenberg (1871 to 1946) was a German physician.
2. Virchow's node is an enlarged left supraclavicular lymph node, most commonly due to metastatic gastric cancer. This nodal station is located where the thoracic duct empties into the left subclavian vein. Gastric metastases are thought to reach this location via emboli in the thoracic duct. Other malignancies in the chest, abdomen, and pelvis can also result in an enlarged Virchow's node. Rudolf Virchow (1821 to 1902) was also a German physician.
3. The Sister Mary Joseph nodule is a palpable umbilical nodule that usually signals metastatic malignancy in the abdomen or pelvis. Sister Mary Joseph (1856 to 1939) was a surgical assistant to Dr. William Mayo, and she noticed the association between encountering an umbilical nodule when prepping the patient's skin for surgery and metastatic intra-abdominal cancer found intraoperatively.

REFERENCES

1. Rubesin SE, Levine MS, Laufer I. Double-contrast upper gastrointestinal radiography: a pattern approach for diseases of the stomach. Radiology 2008;246:33-48.
2. Dicken BJ, Bigam DL, Cass C, Mackey JR, Joy AA, Hamilton SM. Gastric adenocarcinoma: review and considerations for future directions. Ann Surg 2005;24:27-39.
3. Adachi Y, Oshiro T, Okuyama T, et al. A simple classification of lymph node level in gastric carcinoma. Am J Surg 1995;169: 382-385.
4. Siosaki MD, Souza AT. Images in clinical medicine: Virchow's node. N Engl J Med 2013;368:e7.

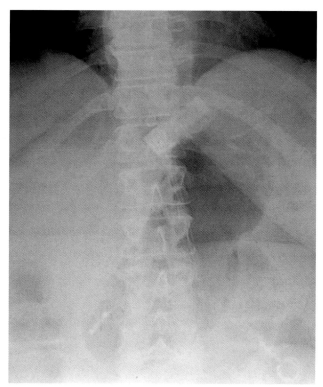

FIGURE 1.19

FINDINGS Abdominal radiograph demonstrates a radiopaque structure overlying the left upper quadrant. Tubing connects this structure to a port overlying the left abdomen.

DIAGNOSIS Adjustable gastric band.

DISCUSSION Adjustable gastric bands are a restrictive method for weight loss. These bands are usually placed laparoscopically and are commonly referred to as "lap bands." When evaluating a lap band at radiography, three features should be assessed: (1) location, (2) shape, and (3) angulation. These features should be assessed on a frontal radiograph. An appropriately positioned band overlies the expected location of the proximal stomach, has a rectangular (rather than circular) shape on a frontal film, and is directed at approximately the 2 o'clock and 8 o'clock positions.

The adjustable gastric band is placed around the proximal stomach approximately 2 cm below the esophagogastric junction, creating a small, approximately 20-mL pouch. These bands are connected via tubing to a port located in the subcutaneous fat of the anterior abdomen. Sterile saline injected via the port results in increased distention of the band. The distended band delays the transit of food from the proximal stomach resulting in a feeling of early satiety and weight loss.

Though practice will vary from surgeon to surgeon, after band placement weight loss may be assessed on a monthly basis. If desired weight loss goals are not being met, the band may be tightened via injection of additional saline either in the surgeon's office or by the surgeon in the fluoroscopy suite with concurrent imaging to evaluate the transit of barium through the level of the band. The band may be increasingly tightened until the patient complains of discomfort.

Indications for the placement of an adjustable gastric band include a body mass index (BMI) (BMI = weight (kg)/height $(m)^2$) of greater than 40 or a BMI between 35 and 40 with medical comorbidities including diabetes or high blood pressure.

Questions for Further Thought

1. What complications may occur following adjustable gastric band placement?
2. How do these complications manifest radiographically?

Reporting Requirements

1. This patient has an adjustable gastric band.
2. The band appears appropriately positioned.

What the Treating Physician Needs to Know

1. Since the band orientation looks normal on this frontal radiograph, it is likely not slipped.
2. If there is clinical concern for band erosion or that the band is too tight, a fluoroscopic contrast study should be performed.
3. If there is clinical concern for a port site complication such as an abscess, ultrasound could evaluate the tissues immediately surrounding the port or CT or MR could be obtained.

Answers

1. Complications of adjustable gastric band placement include band slippage, band erosion, and gastric perforation. Port and tubing complications including infection and disconnected tubing may also occur.
2. Band slippage manifests as an abnormal orientation of the band. Normally the band should appear as a rectangle rather than an "O" on a frontal film as it should be seen on end if appropriately positioned. Additionally, an appropriately positioned band should be directed at the 2 o'clock and 8 o'clock positions. Band erosion manifests as contrast material between the band and the adjacent gastric wall at fluoroscopy. Gastric perforation is indicated by pneumoperitoneum. Inflammatory changes and/or fluid collections around the tubing or port visible at CT may indicate infection. Tubing continuity should be evaluated at radiography and CT.

REFERENCES

1. Pieroni S, Sommer EA, Hito R, Burch M, Tkacz JN. The "O" sign, a simple and helpful tool in the diagnosis of laparoscopic adjustable gastric band slippage. Am J Roentgenol 2010;195:137-141.

2. Blachar A, Blank A, Gavert N, Metzer U, Fluser G, Abu-Abeid S. Laparoscopic adjustable gastric banding surgery for morbid obesity: imaging of normal anatomic features and postoperative gastrointestinal complications. Am J Roentgenol 2007;188: 472-479.

CLINICAL HISTORY *36-year-old woman presents to the emergency department with 2-day history of nausea and vomiting.*

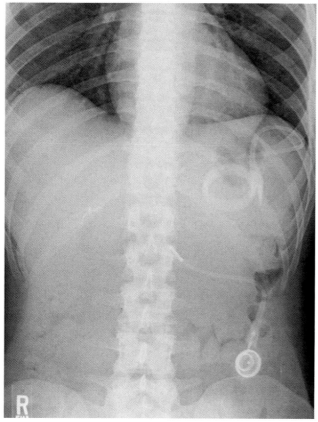

FIGURE 1.20

FINDINGS Abdominal radiograph demonstrates an adjustable gastric band overlying the left upper quadrant. The long axis of the band is oriented perpendicular to the spine and is directed at approximately the 3 o'clock and 9 o'clock positions. The band also has an "O" morphology on this frontal film.

DIFFERENTIAL DIAGNOSIS Appropriately positioned adjustable gastric band, slipped gastric band.

DIAGNOSIS Slipped gastric band.

DISCUSSION When evaluating a gastric band at radiography, three features should be assessed: (1) location, (2) shape, and (3) angulation. These features should be assessed on a frontal radiograph.

First, an appropriately positioned band should overlie the expected location of the proximal stomach. The above band is located too distal, a clue that it is slipped. Second, an appropriately positioned band should appear as a rectangle on a frontal film. A band that has slipped will appear as an "O." This appearance has been referred to as the "O" sign

which indicates a slipped gastric band. The above case illustrates the "O" sign.

Third, the angle formed between an appropriately positioned gastric band and the longitudinal axis of the spine should measure less than approximately 55 degrees on a frontal film. In other words, if one imagines a clock face, a line running along the long axis of the band should be at approximately 2 o'clock and 8 o'clock positions. The above band is oriented at approximately 3 o'clock and 9 o'clock positions, an additional finding that the band has slipped.

Gastric band slippage occurs in approximately 4% to 13% of patients with gastric bands. Two different anatomic explanations for slipped bands have been described. In some cases, the distal stomach herniates retrograde through the band. In other cases, peristalsis pushes the band to a more distal than desired location. In the former scenario, depending on the amount of herniated stomach and the tightness of the band, patients may present with mild obstructive symptoms or may present with complete obstruction and gastric ischemia.

Questions for Further Thought

1. How might a patient with a slipped gastric band present to the emergency department?
2. What is the management of a slipped gastric band?

Reporting Requirements

1. The morphology and angulation of the gastric band indicate that it has slipped.
2. Contact the ordering physician to alert him/her to this unexpected finding.

What the Treating Physician Needs to Know

1. The patient's bariatric surgeon should be consulted for management of this complication.
2. A slipped band should be emergently addressed (see later). Failure to correct a slipped band in a timely manner can result in gastric ischemia.

Answers

1. Patients with slipped bands often present with nausea and vomiting due to a partial or complete gastric obstruction.
2. At a minimum, the band will likely be deflated and reevaluated to determine if deflation relieves the slip. The patient may require emergent surgery to repair or remove the band if there is evidence of complete obstruction and gastric ischemia.

REFERENCES

1. Pieroni S, Sommer EA, Hito R, Burch M, Tkacz JN. The "O" sign, a simple and helpful tool in the diagnosis of laparoscopic adjustable gastric band slippage. Am J Roentgenol 2010;195:137-141.

2. Blachar A, Blank A, Gavert N, Metzer U, Fluser G, Abu-Abeid S. Laparoscopic adjustable gastric banding surgery for morbid obesity: imaging of normal anatomic features and postoperative gastrointestinal complications. Am J Roentgenol 2007;188: 472-479.

CLINICAL HISTORY *43-year-old woman with adjustable gastric band placed 3 years prior experiencing new-onset weight gain but no significant abdominal pain.*

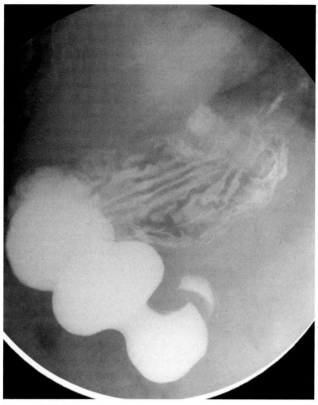

FIGURE 1.21A

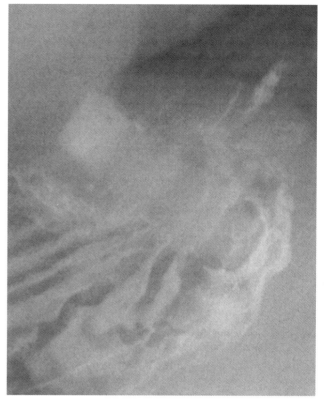

FIGURE 1.21B

FINDINGS Oblique images from an upper GI study (A, B) demonstrate ingested oral contrast material located between the left outer margin of the patient's adjustable gastric band and the gastric wall.

DIFFERENTIAL DIAGNOSIS Eroded gastric band.

DIAGNOSIS Eroded gastric band.

DISCUSSION Adjustable gastric bands (also known as laparotomy bands or lap bands) encircle the outside of the patient's proximal stomach to create an approximately 20-mL gastric pouch. Gastric bands are a restrictive method of weight loss as they result in delayed transit of ingested material through the level of the band, feelings of early satiety, and weight loss.

Since the band should be located outside of the stomach, all ingested contrast material should be located within the confines of the band. Contrast material visible between the outer edge of the band and gastric wall indicates that the band has eroded. Confirmation with EGD is usually performed.

Band erosion occurs in fewer than 10% of patients with adjustable gastric bands. Somewhat surprisingly, patients with eroded gastric bands may be asymptomatic. The only clue to the diagnosis clinically may be new onset weight gain. However, some patients may also experience vague abdominal pain, port site infections, and/or upper abdominal abscesses as a result of band erosion.

Questions for Further Thought

1. What is a proposed mechanism for gastric band erosion?
2. What is the treatment for an eroded gastric band?

Reporting Responsibility

1. Notify the ordering physician that the gastric band appears to have eroded into the stomach.

What the Treating Physician Needs to Know

1. The patient's bariatric surgeon should be consulted.
2. Eroded gastric bands are usually surgically removed (see later).

Answers

1. Pressure necrosis is thought to lead to gastric band erosion.
2. Eroded gastric bands are usually surgically removed given the risk of abscess formation due to gastric perforation.

REFERENCES

1. Hainaux B, Agneessens E, Rubesova E, et al. Intragastric band erosion after laparoscopic adjustable gastric banding for morbid obesity: imaging characteristics of an underreported complication. Am J Roentgenol 2005;184:109-112.
2. Eid I, Birch DW, Sharma AM, Sherman V, Karmali S. Complications associated with adjustable gastric banding for morbid obesity: a surgeon's guide. Can J Surg 2011;54:61-66.

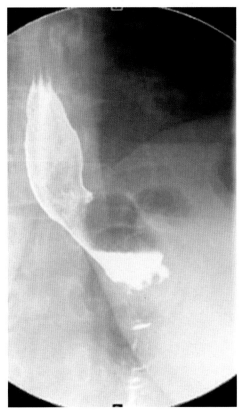

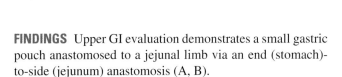

FIGURE 1.22A

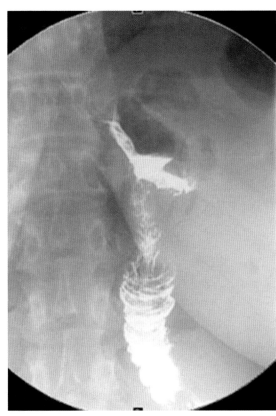

FIGURE 1.22B

FINDINGS Upper GI evaluation demonstrates a small gastric pouch anastomosed to a jejunal limb via an end (stomach)-to-side (jejunum) anastomosis (A, B).

DIFFERENTIAL DIAGNOSIS Adjustable gastric band, Roux-en-Y gastric bypass, sleeve gastrectomy.

DIAGNOSIS Roux-en-Y gastric bypass.

DISCUSSION Roux-en-Y gastric bypass is a weight loss procedure with both a restrictive component and a malabsorptive component. The bariatric surgeon divides the proximal stomach creating an approximately 15- to 20-mL gastric pouch. This small pouch results in a feeling of early satiety and provides the restrictive component of the procedure.

Next, the jejunum is divided approximately 25 to 50 cm beyond the ligament of Treitz. The roux limb of jejunum is anastomosed to the gastric pouch via an end (stomach)-to-side (jejunum) anastomosis. At CT, the roux limb is most commonly located anterior to the transverse colon. Historically, the roux limb was sometimes retrocolic in location, but a retrocolic location was found to have a higher

association with internal hernia and is less commonly performed today.

The excluded portion of the stomach remains in its normal anatomic location and maintains its normal relationship to the duodenum and proximal jejunum. This latter segment of the bowel is referred to as the pancreaticobiliary limb. The excluded stomach and pancreaticobiliary limb are usually not visible at fluoroscopy. The roux limb of jejunum and pancreaticobiliary limb are anastomosed via a jejunojejunostomy which is usually located in the left abdomen. The malabsorptive effect of this surgery occurs because ingested food moves from the gastric pouch into the roux limb bypassing the pancreaticobiliary limb.

At fluoroscopy, a small gastric pouch anastomosed to a jejunal limb is visible. The jejunojejunostomy can be difficult to identify at fluoroscopy. At CT, the gastric pouch, gastrojejunostomy staple line, roux limb (usually passing anterior to the transverse colon), excluded portion of the stomach, and jejunojejunostomy staple line (usually in the left abdomen) are all visible.

By comparison, patients who have undergone adjustable gastric banding will have a radiopaque band overlying the left upper quadrant along with connecting tubing and a port overlying the upper abdomen at radiography. Patients who have undergone sleeve gastrectomy will demonstrate a tubular morphology of the stomach, and the stomach maintains its normal anatomic relationship to the duodenum at fluoroscopy. At CT, the excluded portion of the stomach is not present in patients who have undergone sleeve gastrectomy as it is removed during surgery.

Question for Further Thought

1. What are potential complications of Roux-en-Y gastric bypass surgery?

Reporting Requirements

1. Report that the patient has undergone Roux-en-Y gastric bypass surgery.
2. Assess for complications (see later).

What the Treating Physician Needs to Know

1. The patient has undergone Roux-en-Y gastric bypass surgery.
2. No complication was visible at fluoroscopy.

Answer

1. Potential complications include anastomotic leak (most commonly at the gastrojejunostomy), stomal stenosis (most commonly at the gastrojejunostomy), marginal ulcer (most commonly near the gastrojejunostomy), gastrogastric fistula, and internal hernia.

REFERENCE

1. Scheirey CD, Scholz FJ, Shah PC, Brams DM, Wong BB, Pedrosa M. Radiology of the laparoscopic Roux-en-Y gastric bypass procedure: conceptualization and precise interpretation of results. Radiographics 2006;26:1355-1371.

CLINICAL HISTORY *42-year-old outpatient with abdominal pain, nausea, and vomiting; history of Roux-en-Y gastric bypass surgery 3 years prior.*

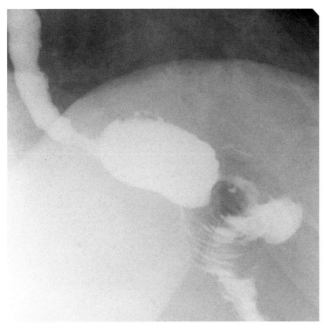

FIGURE 1.23

FINDINGS Upper GI evaluation demonstrates an approximately 2 cm in length segment of marked, fixed narrowing at the site of the gastrojejunostomy. This area did not distend during the study. However, the gastric pouch was distended, and there was delayed clearance of contrast material from the esophagus and gastric pouch. Additionally, an approximately 5-mm ovoid fixed collection of contrast material was seen arising from this area of segmental narrowing.

DIFFERENTIAL DIAGNOSIS Stomal stenosis, marginal ulcer.

DIAGNOSIS Stomal stenosis AND marginal ulcer.

DISCUSSION Stomal stenosis is a relatively common complication following Roux-en-Y gastric bypass surgery occurring in up to 27% of patients. The vast majority of clinically significant stomal stenoses occur at the gastrojejunostomy. Patients may present with abdominal pain, nausea, and vomiting.

Stomal stenosis results from active inflammation at the gastrojejunostomy or chronic fibrosis. Ulcer disease leading to an inflammatory stricture was thought to be the etiology of stomal stenosis in the above patient.

At fluoroscopy, stomal stenosis is suggested when the gastric pouch appears distended, the gastrojejunostomy appears narrowed, and there is delayed transit of contrast material through the gastrojejunostomy.

In the surgical literature, stomal stenosis is defined as clinical signs and symptoms of obstruction along with the inability to pass an 8.5-mm diagnostic endoscope across the gastrojejunostomy.

Questions for Further Thought

1. You are about to perform an upper GI study on an outpatient with abdominal pain and history of prior gastric bypass surgery. List potential etiologies of pain in this patient population.
2. How are stomal stenoses usually treated?

Reporting Requirements

1. This patient has a marginal ulcer along with stomal stenosis.
2. The stomal stenosis is functionally significant as it results in delayed clearance of the contrast column from the esophagus and gastric pouch.

What the Treating Physician Needs to Know

1. This patient would likely benefit from proton pump inhibitors to manage the marginal ulcer.
2. Dilatation may be required to manage the stenosis.

Answers

1. Stomal stenosis, marginal ulcer, and nonobstructed internal hernia are etiologies of abdominal pain encountered in Roux-en-Y gastric bypass patients in the outpatient setting. Anastomotic leaks and obstructed internal hernias are more commonly encountered in inpatients and emergency department patients.
2. Stomal stenoses at the gastrojejunostomy are usually treated by dilatation at endoscopy. Stomal stenoses at the jejunojejunostomy are relatively rare and require surgical correction if symptomatic.

REFERENCES

1. Blachar A, Federle MP, et al. Gastrointestinal complications of laparoscopic Roux-en-Y gastric bypass surgery in patients who are morbidly obese: findings on radiography and CT. Am J Roentgenol 2002;179:1437-1442.
2. Go MR, Muscarella P, Needleman BJ, Cook CH, Melvin WS. Endoscopic management of stomal stenosis after Roux-en-Y gastric bypass. Surg Endosc 2004;18:56-59.

CLINICAL HISTORY *43-year-old woman status post weight loss surgery.*

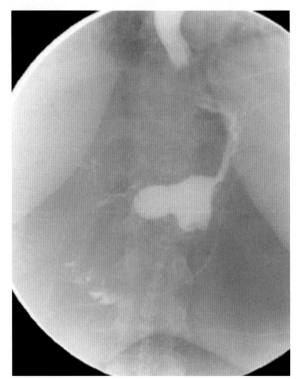

FIGURE 1.24A

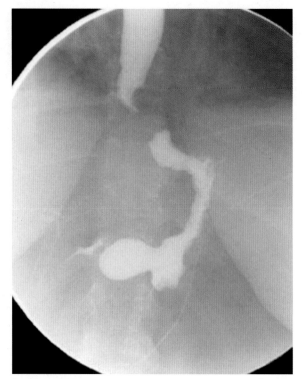

FIGURE 1.24B

FINDINGS Images (A, B) from an upper GI study demonstrate a tubular morphology of the stomach. The stomach maintains its normal anatomic relationship with the duodenum.

DIFFERENTIAL DIAGNOSIS Status post Roux-en-Y gastric bypass surgery, status post sleeve gastrectomy.

DIAGNOSIS Status post sleeve gastrectomy.

DISCUSSION Sleeve gastrectomy is a restrictive form of weight loss surgery whereby the bariatric surgeon removes a large portion of the greater curvature of the stomach. When performing the procedure, a 32- to 46-French bougie is placed through the esophagus into the stomach. This bougie preserves a gastric channel. The surgeon then staples along the bougie and removes the excess stomach.

Sleeve gastrectomy was initially proposed as a surgical weight loss option for people thought to be too high risk for gastric bypass. Initially, sleeve gastrectomy was performed in anticipation of performing a gastric bypass as a second step. However, effective weight loss has been reported in patients undergoing sleeve gastrectomy, and this procedure is now considered to be an effective stand-alone weight loss surgery.

At fluoroscopic imaging, patients who have undergone sleeve gastrectomy may demonstrate a range of morphologies, including a uniform tubular morphology of the stomach, a prominent upper pouch, a prominent lower pouch, and a more dumbbell shape with both upper and lower pouches. An awareness of these different morphologies is important so that a pouch is not misdiagnosed as a leak.

The preferred morphology is a perfect tube. However, sometimes despite the same surgeon using the same technique, different morphologies may result. All of the above-described morphologies are currently considered acceptable. Current investigations are evaluating the relationship between postoperative stomach morphology, weight loss, and gastroesophageal reflux.

Questions for Further Thought

1. What is the reported rate of leak following sleeve gastrectomy?
2. What is the usual CT appearance of a patient who has undergone sleeve gastrectomy?

Reporting Requirements

1. This patient has undergone sleeve gastrectomy.
2. No leak is seen.

What the Treating Physician Needs to Know

1. That the patient has undergone sleeve gastrectomy.
2. There is no evidence of complication such as leak.

Answers

1. Leaks occur at a rate of approximately 2% following sleeve gastrectomy. Overall, complication rates are lower following sleeve gastrectomy as compared with Roux-en-Y gastric bypass.
2. At CT, patients who have undergone sleeve gastrectomy will demonstrate a smaller than usual stomach. This small stomach maintains its normal relationship with the duodenum. A staple line is often visible along the greater curvature of the stomach. The excluded portion of the stomach is discarded and not left in situ in patients undergoing sleeve gastrectomy. By comparison, the excluded portion of the stomach is left in its normal anatomic location in patients undergoing Roux-en-Y gastric bypass procedures.

REFERENCES

1. Goitein D, Goitein O, Feigin A, Zippel D, Papa M. Sleeve gastrectomy: radiologic patterns after surgery. Surg Endosc 2009;23:1559-1563.
2. Shi X, Karmali S, Sharma AM, Birch DW. A review of laparoscopic sleeve gastrectomy for morbid obesity. Obes Surg 2010;20:1171-1177.

CLINICAL HISTORY *54-year-old woman with history of Nissen fundoplication 4 years previously, now with new symptoms of reflux.*

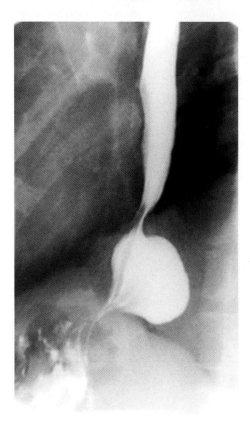

FIGURE 1.25A

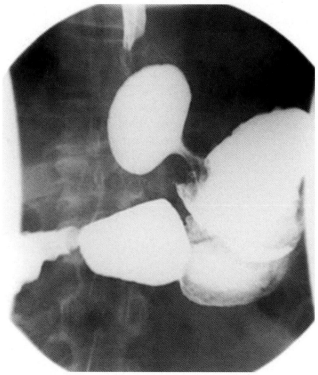

FIGURE 1.25B

FINDINGS Images (A, B) from an upper GI study demonstrate an approximately 2- to 3-cm smooth narrowing located approximately 4 cm below the esophagogastric junction. A distended proximal most stomach is located just above this smooth narrowing. This ballooned proximal most stomach is located above the diaphragm.

DIFFERENTIAL DIAGNOSIS Intact fundoplication, slipped fundoplication.

DIAGNOSIS Slipped fundoplication.

DISCUSSION When evaluating patients who have undergone fundoplication procedures, the following questions should be answered by the fluoroscopy study: (1) Is the wrap intact? (2) Is the wrap in the correct location with respect to the esophagus and diaphragm? (3) Is the wrap too tight?

Fundoplication wraps should be located around the distal esophagus. The above wrap is located approximately 4 cm below the esophagogastric junction and has therefore slipped. Also, the portion of the stomach now located above the wrap is also located above the diaphragm. Not unexpectedly, this patient had recurrent symptoms of GERD.

The term "slipped Nissen" is used to describe the situation in which the Nissen wrap has slipped more inferiorly and is wrapped around the proximal stomach rather than the distal esophagus. As in the above case, a slipped Nissen can be identified by noting contrast material in the esophagus, then in dilated proximal stomach, and then noting a smooth 2- to 3-cm narrowing reflecting the fundoplication wrap located around the stomach rather than the distal esophagus.

Slipped fundoplications are thought to occur most commonly in patients with a shortened esophagus. Chronic scarring caused by GERD can result in a shorter than normal esophagus. When the shortened esophagus retracts back into the thorax following surgery, it can pull the proximal stomach with it causing the fundoplication to slip.

Questions for Further Thought

1. What symptoms may be experienced by a patient with a slipped fundoplication?
2. What is the management of a slipped fundoplication?

Reporting Requirements

1. Report the presence of the fundoplication.

2. Report whether the fundoplication appears intact, in the appropriate location, and if the fundoplication appears too tight.

What the Treating Physician Needs to Know

1. Whether the fundoplication appears intact, in the appropriate location, and if the fundoplication appears too tight.

Answers

1. Patients with slipped fundoplications may present with recurrent symptoms of gastroesophageal reflux.

2. Slipped fundoplications are usually surgically repaired. An esophageal lengthening procedure such as a Collis gastroplasty may be performed as shortened esophagus is thought to predispose to fundoplication slippage. Collis gastroplasty is performed by placing a bougie through the esophagogastric junction and stapling along the stomach side of the esophagogastric junction with resultant creation of a longer esophageal tube.

REFERENCES

1. Canon CL, Morgan DE, Einstein DM, Herts BR, Hawn MT, Johnson LF. Surgical approach to gastroesophageal reflux disease: what the radiologist needs to know. Radiographics 2005;25:1485-1499.

2. Baker ME, Einstein DM, Herts BR, et al. Gastroesophageal reflux disease: integrating the barium esophagram before and after antireflux surgery. Radiology 2007;243:329-339.

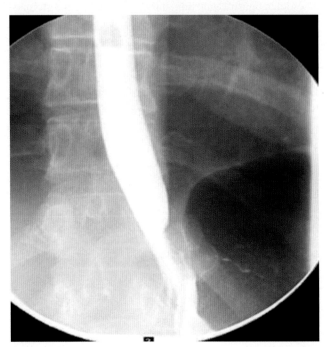

FIGURE 1.26A

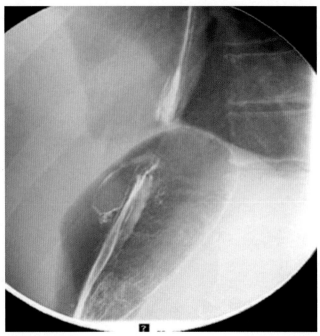

FIGURE 1.26B

FINDINGS Images from a double-contrast upper GI study demonstrate a 3.5-cm smooth mass protruding into the gastric lumen (A). The mass is peripherally etched in contrast material in the second image (B). The mucosal surface of the mass is smooth, and the mass is not causing obstruction.

DIFFERENTIAL DIAGNOSIS Extrinsic compression, mucosal mass, submucosal mass, ulcer.

DIAGNOSIS Submucosal mass (GIST at biopsy).

DISCUSSION The differential diagnosis of a submucosal gastric mass includes benign etiologies (e.g., leiomyoma, schwannoma, neuroma, neurofibroma, lipoma, duplication cyst, and granular cell tumor) and malignant or potentially malignant etiologies (e.g., GIST, lymphoma, metastatic cancer, and glomus tumor). At upper GI, the differential in general cannot be conclusively narrowed beyond "submucosal mass," and tissue sampling is usually required to establish the diagnosis.

As with the esophagus, evaluating whether the gastric mucosa is smooth or irregular can help discriminate between a mucosally based mass and a submucosal or extrinsic process. In the above case, the mucosa is smooth making a mucosally based abnormality such as adenocarcinoma unlikely.

Accurately distinguishing between a mucosal and submucosal or extrinsic mass is important. Mucosal abnormalities will be directly visible at standard endoscopy. By comparison, submucosal masses or areas of extrinsic compression may be difficult to identify with standard endoscopy if the overlying mucosa is smooth. EUS is often better able to locate submucosal masses and areas of extrinsic compression. Additionally, EUS can evaluate the needle trajectory prior to tissue sampling of submucosal masses so that large blood vessels can be avoided.

Evaluating whether contrast material outlines the outer margin of a structure versus fills the central portion of a structure is a helpful way to discriminate between a submucosal mass and an ulcer. As in the above case, contrast material will outline the outside margin of a submucosal mass. By comparison, contrast material will occupy the central portion of an ulcer.

GISTs are the most common submucosal gastric mass. Historically, gastric GISTs were often characterized as leiomyomas. However, newer genetic studies have determined that most of the gastric tumors previously thought to be leiomyomas are actually GISTs. True leiomyomas of the stomach are rare.

Approximately 10% to 30% of GISTs are malignant. All gastric GISTs are assumed to have some malignant potential and are usually removed if the patient is a suitable surgical candidate.

Questions for Further Thought

1. Imagine you are reviewing an upper GI study with a gastric mass and have narrowed the differential diagnosis to a submucosal or extrinsic mass. What imaging test could be performed to narrow the differential?
2. How accurate is endoscopy in distinguishing between submucosal gastric masses and extrinsic compression?

Reporting Requirements

1. Report that this patient has a submucosal gastric mass.
2. Report the approximate size and location of the mass.
3. Report whether or not the mass is obstructing.

What the Treating Physician Needs to Know

1. The patient has a nonobstructing submucosal gastric mass.
2. Tissue sampling (usually performed with EUS) likely will be necessary to establish a diagnosis.

Answers

1. Cross-sectional imaging (CT or MR) is a helpful test to distinguish between submucosal gastric masses and an area of extrinsic compression. Gastric lipomas can be diagnosed at CT or MR based on their homogeneous fat attenuation or signal, but gastric lipomas are rare accounting for <1% of submucosal gastric masses.
2. Endoscopy is 89% to 98% sensitive but only 29% to 64% specific in differentiating intramural lesions from areas of extrinsic compression. EUS has a higher specificity in making this distinction.

REFERENCE

1. Hwang JH, Rulyak SD, Kimmey MB. American Gastroenterological Association Institute technical review on the management of gastric subepithelial masses. Gastroenterology 2006;130:2217-2228.

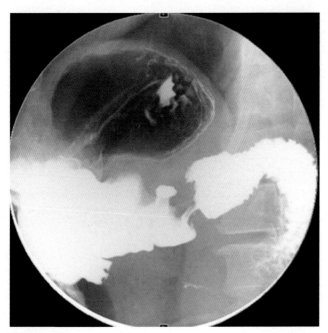

FIGURE 1.27

FINDINGS Image from a double-contrast upper GI study demonstrates an approximately 1.5-cm contrast-filled out-pouching along the distal gastric antrum. There is no evidence of gastric outlet obstruction.

DIFFERENTIAL DIAGNOSIS Diverticulum, ulcer.

DIAGNOSIS Ulcer.

DISCUSSION Active ulcers and diverticula can sometimes be difficult to distinguish during upper GI studies as both will appear as rounded outpouchings of contrast material. Indeed, most acquired gastric diverticula are old ulcer craters. At upper GI, ulcers appear as rounded collections of contrast material. In some cases, the ulcer crater is surrounded by a lucent rim indicating wall edema. If management would change, EGD could be performed to determine if an ulcer is acutely inflamed.

Benign ulcers can sometimes be difficult to distinguish from malignant ulcers. When in doubt, endoscopy with possible tissue sampling should be recommended for further evaluation. Findings that suggest a benign gastric ulcer include a smooth rounded morphology, smooth folds radiating from the ulcer, and a radiolucent line (Hampton line) at the base of the ulcer. By comparison, malignant

ulcers usually occur in areas of necrotic tumor (adenocarcinoma or lymphoma) and are much more irregular in appearance.

The incidence of gastric and duodenal ulcers has decreased in the United States over the last 3 to 4 decades, due in large part to successful medical management. NSAIDs and *Helicobacter pylori* infection are the leading etiologies of peptic ulcer disease. Cessation of NSAID use along with a proton pump inhibitor results in healing of most NSAID-associated ulcers. Triple therapy (proton pump inhibitor along with clarithromycin and amoxicillin to eradicate *H. pylori* infection) results in ulcer healing in most patients with ulcers caused by *H. pylori* infection.

Gastric diverticula most commonly occur in the posterior wall of the gastric fundus, and these fundal diverticula are congenital in origin. By comparison acquired gastric diverticula most commonly occur in the gastric antrum. These acquired diverticula are usually remnants of prior active ulcers as noted above.

Question for Further Thought

1. Are size or location helpful in differentiating benign from malignant ulcers?

Reporting Requirements

1. Report the size and location of the ulcer.
2. Evaluate for complications such as perforation and gastric outlet obstruction.

What the Treating Physician Needs to Know

1. Endoscopy should be performed to evaluate any ulcer that is not clearly benign at upper GI.
2. Most uncomplicated ulcers will heal with medical management.

Answer

1. No. Size and location are not helpful predictors of whether an ulcer is benign or malignant. Morphology is the most helpful feature to distinguish benign from malignant ulcers.

REFERENCES

1. Rubesin SE, Levine MS, Laufer I. Double-contrast upper gastrointestinal radiography: a pattern approach for diseases of the stomach. Radiology 2008;246:33-48.
2. Ramakrishnan K, Salinas RC. Peptic ulcer disease. Am Fam Phys 2007;76:1005-1012.

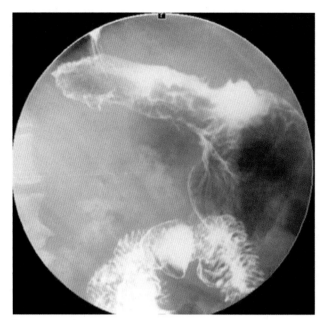

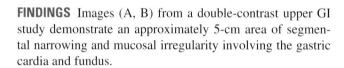

FIGURE 1.28A

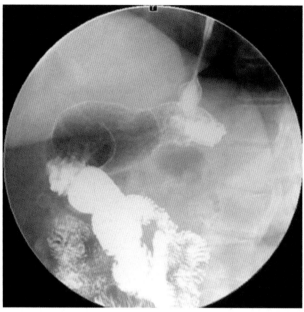

FIGURE 1.28B

FINDINGS Images (A, B) from a double-contrast upper GI study demonstrate an approximately 5-cm area of segmental narrowing and mucosal irregularity involving the gastric cardia and fundus.

DIFFERENTIAL DIAGNOSIS Gastric adenocarcinoma, gastritis, lymphoma.

DIAGNOSIS Gastric adenocarcinoma.

DISCUSSION This degree of mass-like mucosal irregularity is a gastric cancer until proven otherwise. As with the esophagus, determining whether a mass is based in the mucosa, submucosa, or is extrinsic to the stomach can help narrow the differential diagnosis and guide the next diagnostic step (endoscopy for mucosal processes; EUS or cross-sectional imaging [CT or MR] for submucosal or extrinsic processes). Tissue sampling is usually required to reach a definitive diagnosis.

As with the esophagus, mucosal irregularity suggests a mucosa-based process. By comparison, submucosal and extrinsic masses often have a smooth mucosal surface. The mucosal irregularity in the above case indicates that it is a mucosa-based process. Given the severity and relative focality of the abnormality, gastric adenocarcinoma is the most likely diagnosis. Gastritis would not be expected to produce such severe mucosal irregularity.

Lymphoma can also result in mucosal irregularity and may be a multifocal process. Multifocality is therefore a helpful discriminator for gastric lymphoma, a very rare entity. Gastritis can result in relatively subtle mucosal irregularity and

marked fold thickening but would not be expected to cause the amount of mass effect seen in the above case.

Questions for Further Thought

1. What are risk factors for gastric cancer?
2. What is the most common cell type of gastric malignancy?

Reporting Requirements

1. Report that the patient has a large mass occupying much of the gastric cardia and fundus which is highly suspicious for malignancy.
2. Recommend tissue sampling for further evaluation.

What the Treating Physician Needs to Know

1. The findings in this case are highly suspicious for gastric cancer.
2. Endoscopy with tissue sampling should be performed.

Answers

1. Diets rich in preserved and pickled foods, *H. pylori* infection, and atrophic gastritis are thought to increase an individual's risk of developing gastric cancer.
2. About 95% of gastric malignancies are adenocarcinomas.

REFERENCES

1. Rubesin SE, Levine MS, Laufer I. Double-contrast upper gastrointestinal radiography: a pattern approach for diseases of the stomach. Radiology 2008;246:33-48.
2. Dicken BJ, Bigam DL, Cass C, Mackey JR, Joy AA, Hamilton SM. Gastric adenocarcinoma: review and considerations for future directions. Ann Surg 2005;24:27-39.

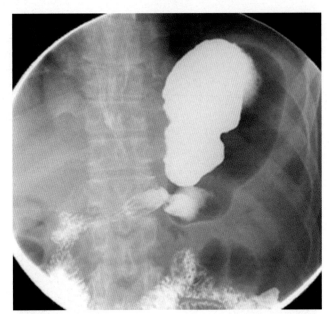

FIGURE 1.29A

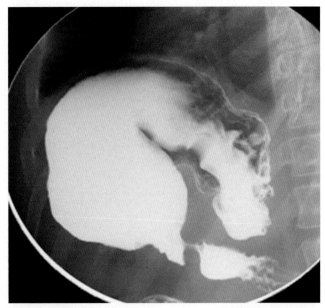

FIGURE 1.29B

FINDINGS Images (A, B) from a double-contrast upper GI study demonstrate the greater curvature of the stomach to be located cranial to the lesser curvature of the stomach. Contrast material readily exits the stomach into the duodenum.

DIFFERENTIAL DIAGNOSIS Mesenteroaxial volvulus, organoaxial volvulus.

DIAGNOSIS Organoaxial volvulus.

DISCUSSION The stomach may rotate along its long axis (organoaxial volvulus), its short axis (mesenteric volvulus), or a combination of both.

Organoaxial volvulus describes the condition whereby the stomach rotates along its long axis with the greater curvature located cranially and the lesser curvature located caudally. In other words, the stomach rotates along a line connecting the esophagogastric junction to the gastric antrum. Organoaxial volvulus is often associated with paraesophageal hiatal hernias. Organoaxial volvulus is more common than mesoaxial volvulus and accounts for approximately two-thirds of gastric volvulus cases.

Mesenteroaxial volvulus occurs much less frequently than organoaxial volvulus. Mesenteroaxial volvulus describes the situation whereby the stomach rotates along its short axis with the antrum located above the esophagogastric junction.

Gastric volvuli are usually surgically repaired. The repair is performed electively if there is no evidence of gastric obstruction. Gastric outlet obstruction would be an indication for emergent repair.

Questions for Further Thought

1. What may be the presenting symptoms of a patient with gastric volvulus?
2. What may be the differential diagnosis suggested by these symptoms?

Reporting Requirements

1. Report that the patient has a gastric volvulus.
2. Report if there is evidence of gastric outlet obstruction.

What the Treating Physician Needs to Know

1. The patient has a gastric volvulus.
2. If there is evidence of gastric outlet obstruction as obstruction is an indication for emergent operative repair.

Answers

1. Patients with gastric volvulus may present with nonspecific symptoms including nausea, vomiting, and abdominal pain. Difficulty passing a nasogastric tube may also indicate a gastric volvulus.
2. Patients with gastric volvulus are often initially thought to have gallstones or peptic ulcer disease.

REFERENCE

1. Peterson CM, Anderson JS, Hara AK, Carenza JW, Menias CO. Volvulus of the gastrointestinal tract: appearances at multimodality imaging. Radiographics 2009;29:1281-1293.

CLINICAL HISTORY *40-year-old woman with abdominal discomfort.*

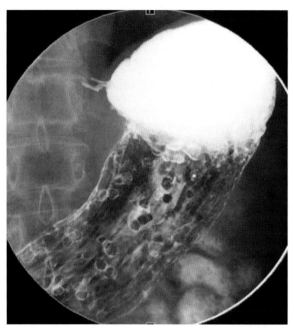

FIGURE 1.30A

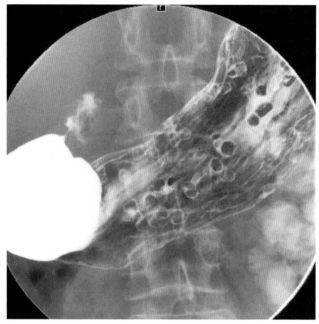

FIGURE 1.30B

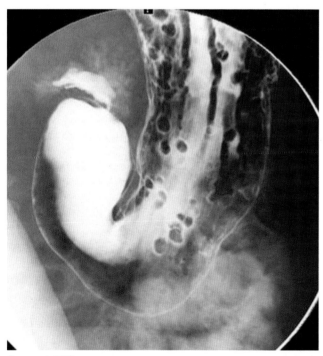

FIGURE 1.30C

FINDINGS Images (A-C) from a double-contrast upper GI study demonstrate innumerable (>20) rounded filling defects in the stomach all measuring approximately 1 cm or less in size. In the primarily air-contrast images (A,B), these rounded structures have a thin rim of barium coating their periphery. In the primarily barium pool image (C), these structures appear as rounded filling defects in the barium pool.

DIFFERENTIAL DIAGNOSIS Polyps, ulcers.

DIAGNOSIS Polyps.

DISCUSSION The abnormality in this case can be characterized as polyps as contrast material is visible outlining the periphery of the numerous lesions in this patient. By comparison, contrast material would pool centrally within gastric ulcers.

Gastric polyps are rare, and when numerous and carpeting the entire stomach as in the above the possibility of a syndrome should be considered. Syndromes associated with gastric polyps include Peutz-Jeghers syndrome, multiple hamartoma syndrome (Cowden disease), familial adenomatous polyposis (FAP) syndrome (Gardner syndrome),

Cronkite-Canada syndrome, and juvenile polyposis syndrome. Alerting the treating physician to the possibility of a syndrome is important as many of these syndromes are associated with increased rates of malignancy and may necessitate additional screening tests.

Facial cutaneous manifestations visible in the fluoroscopy suite may help narrow the differential diagnosis. For example, patients with Peutz-Jeghers syndrome often have pigmented lesions on the lips and mouth. The polyps of Peutz-Jeghers syndrome are hamartomatous and may be found in the stomach, small bowel, or colon.

By comparison, an external marker seen in patients with multiple hamartoma syndrome (Cowden disease) is numerous small hyperkeratoses which most commonly occur on the face. Hamartomas in the setting of Cowden disease may occur anywhere in the GI tract, genitourinary system, bones, and central nervous system. Patients with Cowden disease are thought to be at increased risk for a number of malignancies including breast cancer and thyroid cancer.

The skin findings of Gardner syndrome may be more subtle as small epidermoid cysts may be the only external clue to the diagnosis. Gardner syndrome is a type of FAP syndrome and is characterized by GI polyps, osteomas, and skin tumors. Polyps may occur anywhere in the GI tract, and patients usually undergo prophylactic colectomy due to the high risk of malignant transformation of a colonic polyp and development of colon cancer. Gardner syndrome is also associated with an increased risk of thyroid cancer and mesenteric desmoid tumors.

Skin abnormalities are not commonly associated with juvenile polyposis syndrome though macrocephaly has been described. Juvenile polyps are inflammatory polyps and are most commonly found in the colon and stomach. Patients often present in the second decade of life with anemia and rectal bleeding.

Question for Further Thought

1. What is Cronkite-Canada syndrome?

Reporting Requirements

1. Describe the location, approximate size, and approximate number of polyps.
2. Suggest the possibility of a polyposis syndrome.

What the Treating Physician Needs to Know

1. This patient may have a polyposis syndrome.
2. Several polyposis syndromes are associated with increased risk of malignancy such as familial adenomatous polyposis syndrome which is associated with a high risk of colon cancer.

Answer

1. Cronkite-Canada syndrome is a polyposis syndrome characterized by inflammatory polyps that can occur anywhere along the GI tract, most commonly in the stomach and colon. Thickened gastric folds also may be seen at fluoroscopy. External markers of Cronkite-Canada syndrome include alopecia, absent finger nails and toe nails, and hyperpigmented skin patches.

REFERENCES

1. Gordon R, Laufer I, Kressel HY. Gastric polyps on routine double-contrast examination of the stomach. Radiology 1980;134:27-29.
2. Covarrubias DJ, Huprich JE. Best cases from the AFIP: Juvenile polyposis of the stomach. Radiographics 2002;22:415-420.
3. Buck JL, Harned RK, Lichtenstein JE, Sobin LH. Peutz-Jeghers syndrome. Radiographics 1992;12:365-378.
4. Gold BM, Bagla S, Zarrabi MH. Radiologic manifestations of Cowden disease. Am J Roentgenol 1980;135:385-387.
5. Newman CA, Reuther II WL, Wakabayashi MN, Payette MM, Plavsic BM. Gastrointestinal case of the day. Radiographics 1999;19:546-548.
6. Kilcheski T, Kressel HY, Laufer I, Rogers D. The radiographic appearance of the stomach in Cronkite-Canada syndrome. Radiology 1981;141:57-60.

CLINICAL HISTORY *43-year-old woman with abdominal distention.*

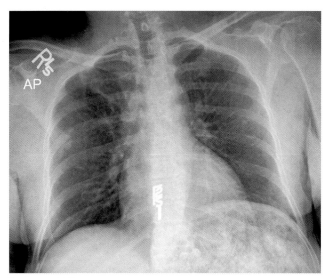

FIGURE 1.31A

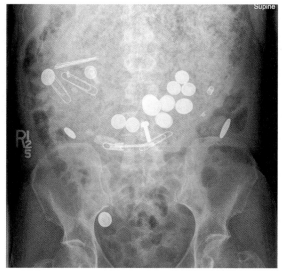

FIGURE 1.31B

FINDINGS Chest and abdominal radiographs (A, B) demonstrate marked distention of the stomach with numerous radiopaque foreign bodies including coins, a zipper, and paper clips. Note the left-sided x-ray marker overlying the distal esophagus. The marker was ingested during the study. Coins also overlie the colon.

DIAGNOSIS Bezoar.

DISCUSSION Bezoar is defined as an accumulation of foreign body material in the GI tract. Phytobezoar refers to a conglomerate of plant material, whereas trichobezoar refers to an accumulation of hair. Phytobezoars are uncommon but tend to occur in patients who have undergone prior gastric surgery such as Billroth II gastroenterostomy. Oranges and persimmons, in particular, are thought to contribute to phytobezoar formation. Trichobezoars tend to occur in female patients who chew and swallow their own hair. The above patient had a psychological disorder resulting in ingestion of numerous foreign bodies.

Abdominal radiographs are relatively insensitive for phyto- and trichobezoars. At CT, phyto- and trichobezoars appear as low-attenuation masses with mottled internal air. Bezoars are often multiple. Therefore, if a GI bezoar is identified at CT, the stomach and the small bowel should be carefully interrogated for additional bezoars.

Surgical gastrostomy with foreign body removal is the usual treatment for gastric bezoars. In addition to the radiopaque foreign bodies visible in the above case, at surgery numerous papers and candy wrappers were also found in the patient's stomach.

The word "bezoar" comes from the Arabic word "bazahr" which means "protection against poison" as in some cultures bezoars found in animals are thought to have medicinal properties.

Question for Further Thought

1. What CT viewing technique can increase the conspicuity of a bezoar?

Reporting Requirement

1. Describe the presence of a very distended stomach containing numerous foreign bodies.

What the Treating Physician Needs to Know

1. This patient has numerous foreign bodies in her stomach.
2. The patient ingested the x-ray marker, and precautions should be taken to prevent the patient from ingesting other foreign bodies during her hospitalization.

Answer

1. Viewing images with a lung or bone window and level can increase the conspicuity of a bezoar.

REFERENCES

1. Ripolles T, Garcia-Aguayo J, Martinez M-J, Gil P. Gastrointestinal bezoars: sonographic and CT characteristics. Am J Roentgenol 2001;177:65-69.
2. http://medical-dictionary.thefreedictionary.com/bezoar. Accessed March 1, 2013.

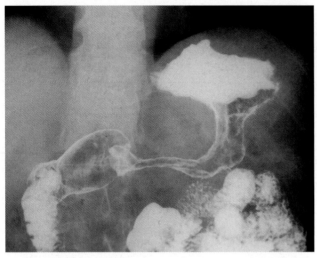

FIGURE 1.32

Metastatic cancer (e.g., lobular breast cancer) and lymphoma can also produce a similar appearance.

Linitis plastica is also sometimes referred to a "leather bottle" stomach. Before glass was widely available, leather bottles were used to store liquids and the shape of these leather bottles was similar to the above gastric shape.

Question for Further Thought

1. How does the prognosis of scirrhous gastric cancer compare with more typical ulcerated or fungating gastric cancers?

Reporting Requirements

1. Report the location of the marked gastric narrowing.
2. Suggest that, given the smoothness of the mucosa, the presumed malignancy may be centered in the submucosa. Therefore, tissue sampling with EUS rather than endoscopy may be necessary.

What the Treating Physician Needs to Know

1. The appearance of the gastric body and antrum is highly suspicious for malignancy.
2. As the pathology appears to be centered in the submucosa, endoscopy may be falsely negative.
3. EUS with tissue sampling may be necessary to target the submucosal layer.

Answer

1. The prognosis of scirrhous gastric cancer is especially poor and is worse than that of more typical gastric cancers. Scirrhous gastric cancers are especially prone to peritoneal metastatic disease.

FINDINGS Double-contrast upper GI study demonstrates marked narrowing of the gastric body and proximal antrum. The gastric mucosa appears relatively smooth.

DIFFERENTIAL DIAGNOSIS Lymphoma, metastatic disease, scirrhous gastric cancer.

DIAGNOSIS Linitis plastica appearance of the stomach due to gastric cancer.

DISCUSSION Diffuse infiltration of the gastric wall is a potential morphology of gastric cancer as in the above case. This type of gastric cancer is also referred to as scirrhous gastric cancer. The rigid, narrowed morphology of the stomach is referred to as linitis plastica and results from extensive fibrosis of the gastric submucosa. When malignant cells are confined primarily to the submucosa, the mucosal surface may appear smooth as above. At endoscopy, the mucosa may also appear relatively normal even in patients with advanced disease as above. As the mucosa may appear normal at endoscopy, EUS is often necessary to guide tissue sampling.

REFERENCES

1. Park M-S, Ha HK, Choi BS, et al. Scirrhous gastric carcinoma: endoscopy versus upper gastrointestinal radiography. Radiology 2004;231:421-426.
2. Levine MS, Pantongrag-Brown L, Aguilera NS, Buck JK, Buetow PC. Non-Hodgkin lymphoma of the stomach: a cause of linitis plastica. Radiology 1996;201:375-378.

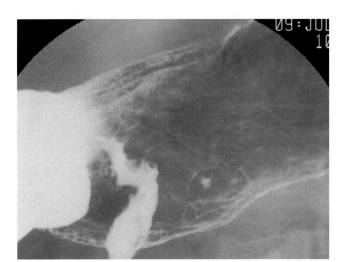

FIGURE 1.33A

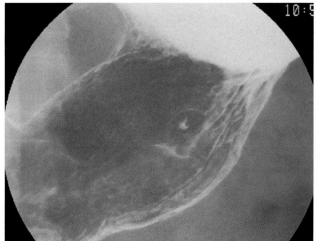

FIGURE 1.33B

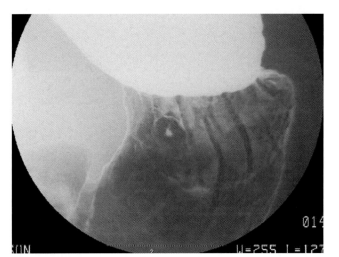

FIGURE 1.33C

FINDINGS Images (A–C) from a double-contrast upper GI study demonstrate several approximately 2-cm elevated lesions with smooth margins and a small amount of central ulceration.

DIFFERENTIAL DIAGNOSIS Lymphoma, metastatic disease.

DIAGNOSIS Metastatic disease (metastatic melanoma).

DISCUSSION The above masses are most likely submucosal in location given their predominantly smooth mucosal surface. When multiple gastric submucosal masses are identified, the differential diagnosis includes lymphoma and metastatic disease.

Melanoma is the most common tumor to metastasize to the stomach followed by lung cancer and breast cancer. In one series, 65% of gastric metastases were solitary and 35% were multiple.[1]

Question for Further Thought

1. What would be an additional differential diagnostic consideration in an HIV-positive patient with multiple submucosal masses?

Reporting Requirements

1. Describe the presence of multiple gastric masses that are suspicious for metastatic disease or lymphoma.
2. Describe the location of the masses to aid the endoscopist in tissue sampling.

What the Treating Physician Needs to Know

1. Findings are suspicious for malignancy.
2. Tissue sampling likely will be necessary to establish the diagnosis.

Answer

1. Kaposi's sarcoma can also appear as multiple submucosal masses with central ulceration.

REFERENCES

1. Oda, Kondo H, Yamao T, et al. Metastatic tumors to the stomach: analysis of 54 patients diagnosed at endoscopy and 347 autopsy cases. Endoscopy 2001;33:507-510.
2. Kanthan R, Sharanowski K, Senger JL, Fesser J, Chibbar R, Kanthan SC. Uncommon mucosal metastases to the stomach. World Jnl Surg Oncol 2009;7:62.
3. Rubesin SE, Levine MS, Laufer I. Double-contrast upper gastrointestinal radiography: a pattern approach for diseases of the stomach. Radiology 2008;246:33-48.

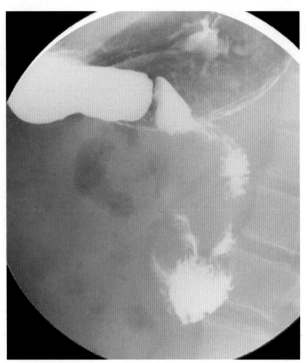
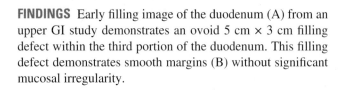

FIGURE 1.34A

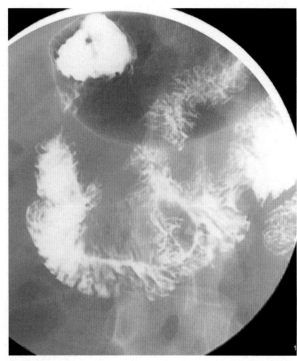

FIGURE 1.34B

FINDINGS Early filling image of the duodenum (A) from an upper GI study demonstrates an ovoid 5 cm × 3 cm filling defect within the third portion of the duodenum. This filling defect demonstrates smooth margins (B) without significant mucosal irregularity.

DIFFERENTIAL DIAGNOSIS Adenocarcinoma, submucosal mass.

DIAGNOSIS Submucosal mass (lipoma).

DISCUSSION Evaluation of the mucosal surface of a duodenal mass can help narrow the differential diagnosis. For example, mucosal irregularity favors a mucosally based process such as adenocarcinoma. By comparison, a smooth mucosal surface as in the above case favors a submucosal mass.

At fluoroscopy, duodenal lipomas appear as well-circumscribed masses. These masses may be compressible in thin patients. At CT, the diagnosis of a lipoma can be made with confidence based on the detection of a homogeneous fat attenuation mass.

Lipomas are often asymptomatic. However, lipomas can ulcerate and be a source of bleeding. The lipoma in the above patient was ulcerated and bleeding and was believed to be the etiology of the patient's anemia.

Question for Further Thought

1. What technique (endoscopy or EUS) is preferred for tissue sampling of submucosal masses?

Reporting Requirement

1. Describe the presence of a 5-cm submucosal mass in the third portion of the duodenum.

What the Treating Physician Needs to Know

1. EUS with tissue sampling should be considered to establish the diagnosis.
2. Alternatively, CT could be performed to distinguish between an entirely fat attenuation lipoma and a soft-tissue mass.

Answer

1. EUS is the preferred technique for tissue sampling of submucosal masses. Submucosal masses that do not disrupt the mucosa may be difficult to localize without ultrasound guidance. Ultrasound also allows for evaluation for large blood vessels in the needle trajectory prior to tissue sampling.

REFERENCE

1. Thompson WM. Imaging and findings of lipomas of the gastrointestinal tract. Am J Roentgenol 2005;184:1163-1171.

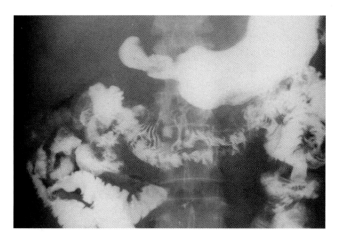

FIGURE 1.35A

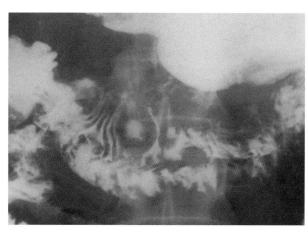

FIGURE 1.35B

FINDINGS Images (A, B) from an upper GI study demonstrate two small areas of contrast pooling in the transverse duodenum with surrounding relative lucency resulting in a "bulls-eye" appearance. These lesions are nonobstructing.

DIFFERENTIAL DIAGNOSIS GIST, lymphoma, metastatic disease.

DIAGNOSIS Metastatic disease (melanoma).

DISCUSSION As with the esophagus and stomach, determining if a lesion is centered in the mucosa, submucosa, or external to the duodenum can help narrow the differential diagnosis. For example, mucosal-based malignant lesions are most commonly adenocarcinomas, are usually ill-defined, and markedly distort the duodenal fold pattern. By comparison, submucosal tumors may appear more well defined and will be less disruptive to the duodenal fold pattern. Lesions extrinsic to the duodenum also often result in preservation of the duodenal fold pattern.

The two ulcerated lesions in the above case have a broad differential though their multiplicity favors metastases. Tissue sampling was ultimately necessary to establish a diagnosis of metastatic melanoma.

Metastases to the duodenum are rare. Melanoma is the tumor that most often metastases to the GI tract. Approximately 2% of melanoma patients have clinically detected GI tract metastases though at autopsy up to 60% of patients with diffuse melanosis have GI tract involvement. Case reports of other primary malignancies such as lung cancer metastasizing to the duodenum have also been described.

GISTs most commonly occur in the stomach and rarely occur in the duodenum. These submucosal tumors typically appear as well-circumscribed masses, often with central ulceration. Primary duodenal lymphoma is also a rare tumor that can appear as a duodenal mass with central ulceration. Most duodenal lymphomas are non-Hodgkin lymphomas.

Question for Further Thought

1. How could tissue be obtained in the above case to establish a diagnosis?

Reporting Requirements

1. Describe the size and location of the above lesions.
2. Report whether the lesions are obstructing.

What the Treating Physician Needs to Know

1. The location of the lesions as this information will be helpful to plan tissue sampling.
2. If there is evidence of obstruction. For example, in patients with obstructing lesions nutritional bypass options such as jejunal tube feeds may be necessary until the obstructing lesions can be addressed.

Answer

1. These lesions could likely be reached with EGD which usually can access most of the duodenum. It is important to characterize based on imaging whether a lesion will likely be visible via EGD or if EUS will be necessary. For example, lesions that disrupt the mucosa like the two ulcerated masses in the above case should be

visible with a camera from the lumen of duodenum and therefore accessible to tissue sampling. By comparison, a submucosal mass that does not distort the mucosa may appear as a focal, mucosal-covered bulge at EGD. Endoscopists generally biopsy such submucosal masses with EUS rather than EGD as EUS allows for visualization of major blood vessels prior to tissue sampling so that such vessels can be avoided.

REFERENCES

1. Benedeto-Stojanov DA, Nagorni AV, Zivkovic VV, Milanovic JR, Stojanov DA. Metastatic melanoma of the stomach and the duodenum. Arch Oncol 2006;14:60-61.

2. Kim H-C, Lee JM, Son KR, et al. Gastrointestinal stromal tumors of the duodenum: CT and barium study findings. Am J Roentgenol 2004;183:415-419.

3. Chestovich PJ, Schiller G, Sasu S, Hiatt JR. Duodenal lymphoma: a rare and morbid tumor. Am Surg 2007;73:1057-1062.

CLINICAL HISTORY *87-year-old woman with abdominal pain.*

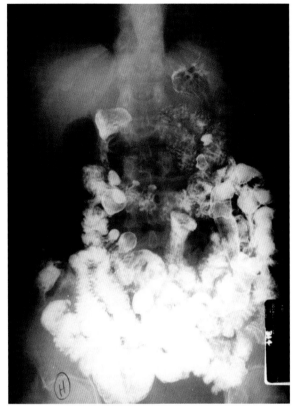

FIGURE 1.36A

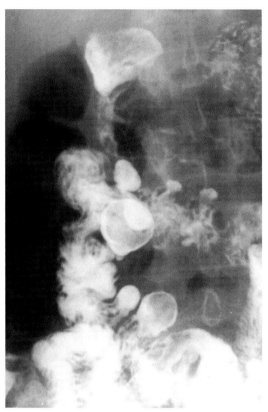

FIGURE 1.36B

FINDING Overhead image (A) and magnified image (B) from a small bowel follow-through demonstrate numerous well-circumscribed outpouchings of contrast material arising from the jejunum and ileum.

DIFFERENTIAL DIAGNOSIS Diverticula, ulcers.

DIAGNOSIS Diverticula.

DISCUSSION Jejunal diverticula are detected at barium studies in approximately 2% of patients, and ileal diverticula are even less common. Diverticula can be distinguished from ulcers by their round shape, smooth margin, and narrow neck.

Diverticula can be categorized as congenital or acquired, pulsion or traction, and true or pseudodiverticula. Congenital diverticula are diverticula like a Meckel diverticulum that are present at birth. Acquired diverticula develop over time. Pulsion diverticula result when, for example, increased intraluminal pressures cause the mucosal lining of a bowel segment to protrude through an area of bowel wall weakness. By comparison, traction diverticula occur when an area of inflammation or scarring adjacent to the bowel results in tethering and focal dilation of a bowel segment. True diverticula contain all layers of bowel wall, whereas pseudodiverticula only contain some layers of the bowel wall.

Small bowel diverticula are acquired pulsion pseudodiverticula. These diverticula occur when the mucosal lining of small bowel protrudes through a weakness in the small bowel wall, usually along the mesenteric side. Small bowel diverticula are pseudodiverticula as their walls are composed of only mucosal and submucosal layers.

Question for Further Thought

1. Are jejunal and ileal diverticula more readily visualized at small bowel follow-through or CT?

Reporting Requirement

1. Describe the presence of numerous jejunal and ileal diverticula.

What the Treating Physician Needs to Know

1. Jejunal and ileal diverticula are usually asymptomatic.
2. Jejunal and ileal diverticula can result in abdominal pain if they become inflamed.
3. Bacterial overgrowth in small bowel diverticula has been posited as an etiology of unexplained diarrhea.

Answer

1. Jejunal and ileal diverticula are more easily seen at fluoroscopic small bowel follow-through than CT. In one study of 28 patients with jejunal and ileal diverticula seen at small bowel follow-through, diverticula were only identified prospectively at CT in 7% of the same patients and retrospectively at CT in 75% of the patients.

REFERENCES

1. Jenkinson EL. Diverticula of the small bowel. Radiology 1929;12:100-105.
2. Fintelmann F, Levine MS, Rubesin SE. Jejunal diverticulosis: findings on CT in 28 patients. Am J Roentgenol 2008;190:1286-1290.

CLINICAL HISTORY *42-year-old woman with abdominal discomfort.*

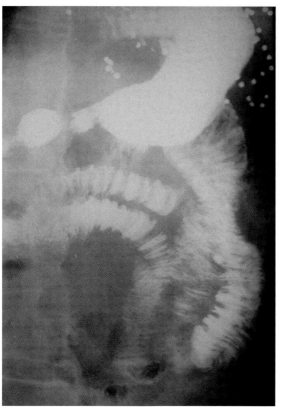

FIGURE 1.37A

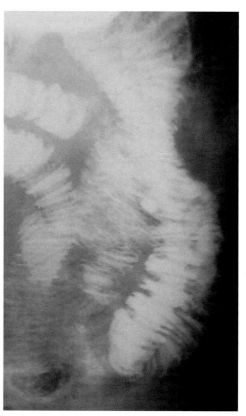

FIGURE 1.37B

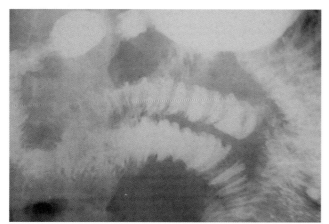

FIGURE 1.37C

FINDINGS Overhead image (A) and magnified views (B, C) from a small bowel follow-through study demonstrate small bowel folds that appear thickened and abnormally close together. Incidentally noted shrapnel from a shotgun overlying the left upper quadrant.

DIFFERENTIAL DIAGNOSIS Amyloid, mechanical small bowel obstruction, scleroderma.

DIAGNOSIS Scleroderma.

DISCUSSION Scleroderma is a connective tissue disorder characterized by extensive deposition of fibrous tissue and muscular atrophy. The closely spaced small bowel folds in the above case are characteristics of scleroderma. Patients with scleroderma may also demonstrate small bowel sacculations due to areas of asymmetric fibrosis, dilated small bowel loops, and delayed small bowel transit times.

Scleroderma can be characterized as localized scleroderma which only involves the skin. By comparison, systemic scleroderma can also involve the GI tract, lungs, heart, and kidneys. The esophagus is the most commonly involved segment of the GI tract. Esophageal findings of scleroderma include a patulous and aperistaltic distal esophagus, often with gastroesophageal reflux. The small intestine is the second most commonly involved segment of the GI tract.

Question for Further Thought

1. What skin findings may be seen in patients with scleroderma?

Reporting Requirement

1. The above appearance of the small bowel is highly suggestive of scleroderma.

What the Treating Physician Needs to Know

1. Patients with scleroderma and small bowel involvement may experience discomfort due to delayed small bowel transit.

2. Delayed small bowel transit may also lead to bacterial overgrowth and problems with malabsorption and diarrhea.

Answer

1. Patients with scleroderma may demonstrate tight skin. This finding may be especially noticeable around the mouth, and the mouth may appear small. Skin tightening involving the finger tips can result in a waxy appearance.

REFERENCE

1. Levine MS, Rubesin SE, Laufer I. Pattern approach for diseases of mesenteric small bowel on barium studies. Radiology 2008;249:445-460.

CLINICAL HISTORY *33-year-old man with abdominal pain 1 month following bone marrow transplant.*

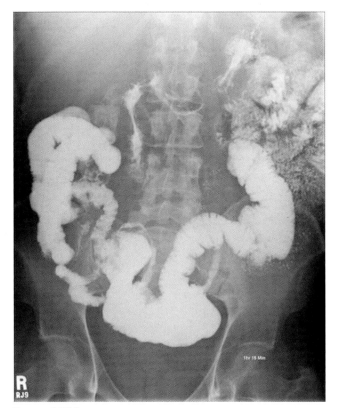

FIGURE 1.38A

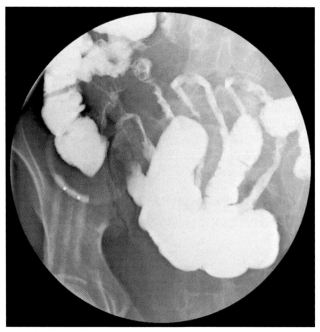

FIGURE 1.38B

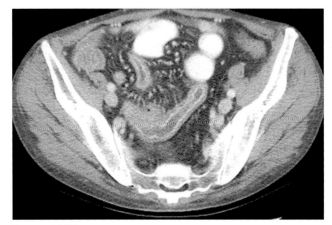

FIGURE 1.38C

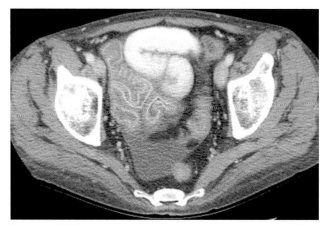

FIGURE 1.38D

FINDINGS Overhead (A) and spot fluoroscopic (B) images from a small bowel follow-through study demonstrate several abnormal loops of ileum in the lower abdomen. These abnormal loops demonstrate luminal narrowing which is indirect evidence of bowel wall edema. CT images obtained after administration of intravenous and oral contrast material (C, D) demonstrate corresponding markedly abnormal small bowel wall thickening as well as small volume free fluid. Note the relative hyperemia of the small bowel mucosa and the lower attenuation of the remainder of the bowel wall.

DIFFERENTIAL DIAGNOSIS Infectious, ischemic, or inflammatory enteritis.

DIAGNOSIS Graft-versus-host disease (GVHD).

DISCUSSION GVHD occurs in bone marrow transplant recipients when donor lymphocytes attack the recipient's cells. GVHD most commonly affects the skin, liver, and GI tract. Skin involvement in the form of a rash or itchy skin is the most common and usually the first manifestation of GVHD. GI involvement in the absence of skin involvement is rare.

For patients with GI GVHD, symptoms will depend on the portion of the intestinal tract involved. For example, patients with proximal involvement (e.g., esophagus or stomach) may experience dysphagia, nausea, and vomiting. By comparison, patients with small bowel or colon involvement may experience abdominal pain and diarrhea.

At fluoroscopy, small bowel involvement with GVHD may manifest as segmental areas of luminal narrowing as in the above case. At CT, the marked mucosal hyperemia and surrounding low attenuation in the bowel wall in the above case is an example of the "halo sign" that is sometimes seen with GVHD. Adjacent fluid may also be evident at CT. Small bowel involvement is more common than large bowel involvement, and discontinuous bowel segments may be involved.

Question for Further Thought

1. What is the usual treatment for GVHD?

Reporting Requirement

1. Describe the presence and distribution of abnormal bowel wall thickening.

What the Treating Physician Needs to Know

1. The distribution of abnormal bowel wall thickening as this information will help guide tissue sampling.
2. If there is evidence of bowel obstruction or perforation.

Answer

1. GVHD is usually treated with immunosuppressive drugs such as steroids and methotrexate. As the imaging appearance of GVHD is often difficult to distinguish from an infectious enteritis, patients usually undergo tissue sampling to establish a definitive diagnosis prior to treatment.

REFERENCES

1. Coy DL, Ormazabal A, Godwin JD, Lalani T. Imaging evaluation of pulmonary and abdominal complications following hematopoietic stem cell transplantation. Radiographics 2005;25: 305-317.
2. Kalantari BN, Mortele KJ, Cantisani V, et al. CT features with pathologic correlation of acute gastrointestinal graft-versus-host disease after bone marrow transplantation in adults. Am J Roentgenol 2003;181:1621-1625.

CLINICAL HISTORY *34-year-old man with abdominal pain.*

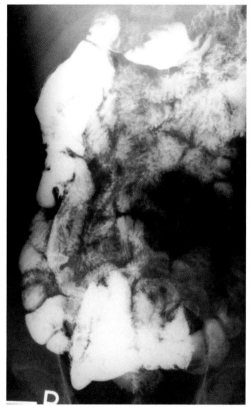

FIGURE 1.39A

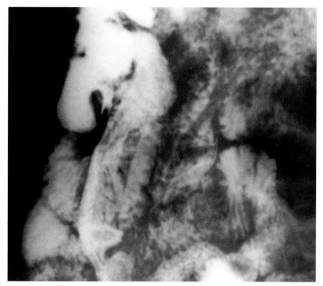

FIGURE 1.39B

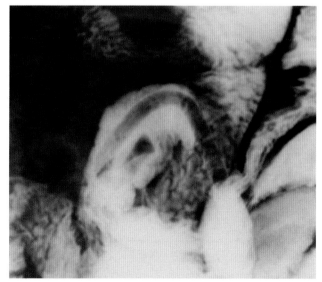

FIGURE 1.39C

FINDINGS Overhead image from small bowel follow-through (A) demonstrates several tubular filling defects including in distal small bowel loops in the right abdomen. Also note the tubular filling defect in a loop of small bowel in the mid-lower abdomen. Magnified image (B) demonstrates tubular somewhat vertically oriented filling defects in the distal small bowel and terminal ileum. Additional magnified image (C) demonstrates a tubular filling defect with a central linear area of contrast material.

DIFFERENTIAL DIAGNOSIS Ingested foreign bodies, parasite infestation.

DIAGNOSIS Parasite infection (ascariasis).

DISCUSSION The differential diagnosis for multiple linear filling defects within small bowel loops includes ingested foreign bodies and parasite infestation with intraluminal worms. Contrast material visible within the intestinal tract of the worm in image C is diagnostic of parasite infestation.

   Though relatively rare in the United States, *Ascaris lumbricoides* infection is relatively common worldwide affecting up to 25% of the world's population. *Ascaris* eggs are transmitted in feces and ingested by human hosts via contaminated food and water. Larvae hatched from ingested eggs migrate via the bloodstream to the lungs where they can produce fever, productive cough, and opacities at chest radiography. The worms then climb out of the lungs, up the trachea, are then swallowed, and may live for up to a year in human hosts growing up to 35 cm in length.

Ascaris worms can also find their way into other portions of the GI tract such as the biliary duct and pancreatic duct and can result in acute cholecystitis and pancreatitis. Surprisingly, patients with ascariasis infestation may be relatively asymptomatic with no or vague abdominal pain. White blood cell count is normal though eosinophilia is usually present. Large clusters of worms may result in a mechanical small bowel obstruction.

Other parasitic worms that may involve the GI tract include *Schistosoma*, *Strongyloides*, *Taenia solium*, *Echinococcus*, *Toxocara*, *Angiostrongylus*, and *Trichuris*. *Ascaris* worms are the largest worms and are the most readily visible at imaging. *Trichuris* worms may be visible as tiny curvilinear filling defects. The other listed worms are usually too small to resolve at imaging but may cause secondary findings such as bowel wall thickening and focal lesions in the solid abdominal organs.

Question for Further Thought

1. What is the usual treatment for ascariasis infestation?

Reporting Requirements

1. Describe the presence of intestinal worms.
2. Evaluate for secondary bowel obstruction.

What the Treating Physician Needs to Know

1. This patient has ascariasis infestation of the intestines.
2. There is no bowel obstruction.

Answer

1. A single 400-mg dose of albendazole is usually curative.

REFERENCES

1. Rodriguez EJ, Gama MA, Ornstein SM, Anderson WD. Ascariasis causing small bowel volvulus. Radiographics 2003;23: 1291-1293.
2. Bahu MGS, Baldisseroto M, Custodio CM, Gralha C, Mangili AR. Hepatobiliary and pancreatic complications of ascariasis in children: a study of seven cases. J Ped Gastroenterol Nutr 2001;33:271-275.
3. Ortega CD, Ogawa NY, Rocha MS, et al. Helminthic diseases in the abdomen: an epidemiologic and radiologic overview. Radiographics 2010;30:253-267.

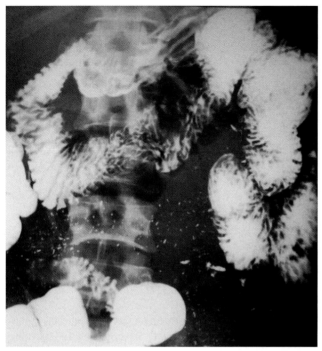

FIGURE 1.40A

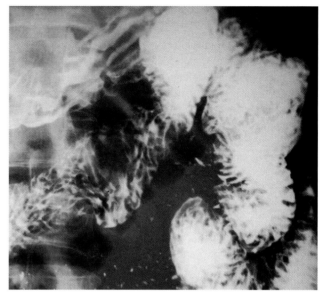

FIGURE 1.40B

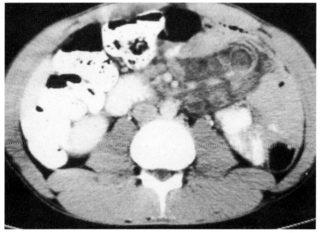

FIGURE 1.40C

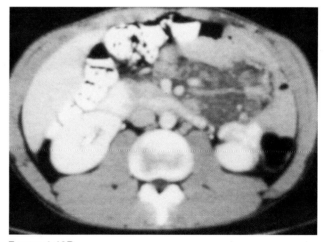

FIGURE 1.40D

FINDINGS Overhead (A) and magnified (B) images from a small bowel follow-through study demonstrate nodular small bowel fold thickening in the left upper quadrant. Numerous low-attenuation lymph nodes are seen in the small bowel mesentery (C, D).

DIFFERENTIAL DIAGNOSIS OF IRREGULAR FOLD THICKENING
Amyloidosis, intestinal lymphangiectasia, *Mycobacterium avium-intracellulare* (MAI), Whipple disease.

DIAGNOSIS Whipple disease.

DISCUSSION Whipple disease is due to infection with *Tropheryma whipplei*. Arthralgias and diarrhea are the most common symptoms as this bacteria targets small bowel and joints. Other less frequent findings include endocarditis and neurologic symptoms including dementia as the bacteria also targets heart valves and the central nervous system.

At imaging, nodular small bowel fold thickening may be visible. Low-attenuation lymph nodes result from lymphatic obstruction by the bacteria, and the combination of nodular fold thickening and low-attenuation lymph nodes is characteristic of Whipple disease.

If untreated, Whipple disease is universally fatal. Treatment is antibiotic therapy including tetracycline. Extensive antibiotic therapy including a 1- to 2-year course of daily trimethoprim–sulfamethoxazole may be necessary to clear recurrent infections.

MAI can be indistinguishable from Whipple disease at imaging. MAI involvement of the GI tract most commonly occurs in patients with AIDS. By comparison, Whipple disease is an extremely rare disease that can occur in otherwise healthy individuals.

Other processes that can produce irregular small bowel fold thickening include amyloidosis and intestinal lymphangiectasia. GI amyloidosis occurs in individuals with systemic amyloid and appears as irregular fold thickening often with patulous loops and delayed small bowel transit time. Intestinal lymphangiectasia refers to dilation of intestinal lymphatic channels and may be congenital or acquired (e.g., due to fibrosis or obstructing tumor).

Question for Further Thought

1. How is Whipple disease diagnosed?

Reporting Requirement

1. Describe the presence of irregular small bowel fold thickening and low-attenuation lymph nodes.

What the Treating Physician Needs to Know

1. Irregular small bowel fold thickening and low-attenuation lymph nodes may be due to Whipple disease or MAI infection.
2. Clinical correlation can help narrow the differential as Whipple disease may occur in otherwise healthy individuals, whereas GI MAI infection most commonly occurs in AIDS patients.
3. Histologic analysis of small bowel biopsy specimens may be necessary to establish the diagnosis.

Answer

1. Whipple disease is diagnosed by identifying inclusions in small bowel biopsy specimens.

REFERENCES

1. Fenollar F, Puechal X, Raoult D. Whipple's disease. N Engl J Med 2007;356:55-66.
2. Levine MS, Rubesin SE, Laufer I. Pattern approach for diseases of mesenteric small bowel on barium studies. Radiology 2008;249:445-460.

CASE 1.41

CLINICAL HISTORY *31-year-old woman with weight loss and diarrhea.*

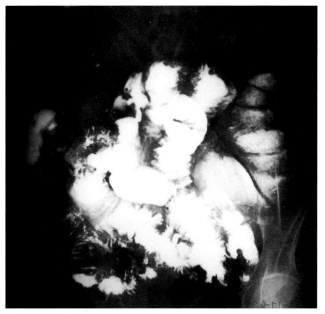

FIGURE 1.41A

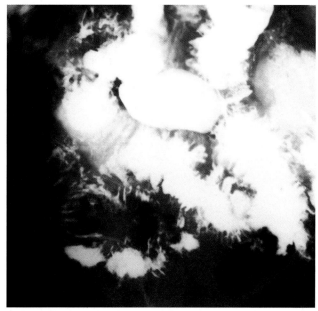

FIGURE 1.41B

FINDINGS Overhead image (A) and magnified image (B) from small bowel follow-through demonstrate numerous bowel folds in the ileum.

DIFFERENTIAL DIAGNOSIS Celiac disease, malabsorption due to pancreatic insufficiency, normal bowel-fold pattern.

DIAGNOSIS Celiac disease.

DISCUSSION In normal subjects, more absorption occurs in the jejunum when compared with the ileum. This difference in absorption is reflected by the increased number of bowel wall folds (and resultant larger surface area for absorption) in the jejunum when compared with the ileum.

By comparison, individuals with malabsorption disorders often develop an increased number of ileal folds as the body responds by trying to increase the available surface area for absorption, the so-called jejunization of ileal loops finding. The identification of an increased number of ileal folds is a generic finding in patients with malabsorption. For example, patients with pancreatic insufficiency due to chronic pancreatitis or cystic fibrosis as well as patients with celiac disease may demonstrate an increased number of ileal folds.

An additional finding often seen in patients with celiac disease (though not well demonstrated in the above case) is a diminished number of or absent jejunal folds. Celiac disease

is an autoimmune disease that results in an inflammatory response to gluten. Histopathologic changes seen at small bowel biopsy include inflammatory changes and villous atrophy. Histopathologic changes are usually most severe in the duodenum and jejunum. Celiac disease is diagnosed by the identification of characteristic histopathologic changes at small bowel biopsy and symptomatic relief with a gluten-free diet.

Other findings that have been described in the setting of malabsorption include flocculation of the barium contrast column, bowel distention, and slow transit. Flocculation refers to a clump-like appearance of ingested barium within small bowel loops and reflects precipitation of barium. This precipitation is thought to occur in patients with malabsorption due to an abnormally large amount of fluid within the small bowel lumen. However, flocculation is a nonspecific finding and can occur in varying amounts depending on the volume and rate of contrast material ingested as well as the consistency of the barium ingested. Bowel distention and slow transit in isolation are also nonspecific findings.

Questions for Further Thought

1. How might patients with celiac disease present?
2. How is celiac disease treated?
3. What are potential complications of untreated or treatment refractory celiac disease?

Reporting Requirement

1. Describe the presence of an abnormal number of ileal folds, a finding indicating malabsorption.

What the Treating Physician Needs to Know

1. A variety of conditions including celiac disease and pancreatic insufficiency can result in this malabsorptive pattern.
2. Correlation with clinical variables and other underlying medical conditions is necessary to determine the etiology of malabsorption.
3. Small bowel biopsy may be necessary to establish a definitive diagnosis.

Answers

1. Patients often present with nonspecific abdominal pain and diarrhea. Celiac disease may affect up to 1 in 200 adults but is thought to often go undiagnosed in part due to the nonspecific nature of symptoms.
2. Strict adherence to a gluten-free diet is the first-line treatment for celiac disease.
3. Potential long-term complications of untreated or treatment-refractory celiac disease include small bowel ulceration, lymphoma, and adenocarcinoma.

REFERENCES

1. Weizman Z, Stringer DA, Dunrie PR. Radiologic manifestations of malabsorption: a nonspecific finding. Pediatrics 1984;74:530-533.
2. Kumar P, Bartram CI. Relevance of the barium follow-through examination in the diagnosis of adult celiac disease. Gastrointest Radiol 1979;4:285-289.
3. Scholz FJ, Afnan J, Behr SC. CT findings in adult celiac disease. Radiographics 2011;31:977-992.
4. Soyer P, Boudiaf M, Fargeaudou Y, et al. Celiac disease in adults: evaluation with MDCT enteroclysis. Am J Roentgenol 2008;191:1483-1492.

CLINICAL HISTORY *23-year-old man with chronic constipation.*

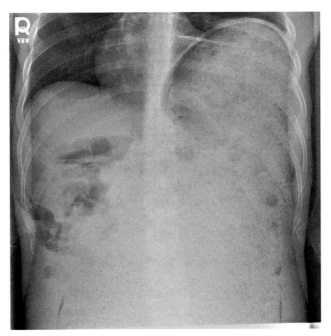

FIGURE 1.42A

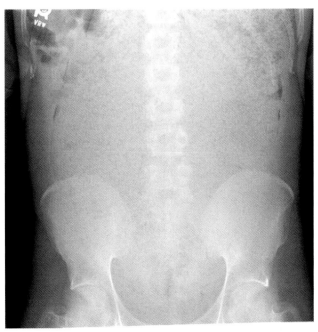

FIGURE 1.42B

FINDINGS Two abdominal radiographs (A, B) demonstrate marked distention of the patient's descending colon, sigmoid colon, and rectum that are filled with stool. The colon measures up to 26 cm in transverse dimension and fills the patient's abdomen and pelvis. Note the minimal gaseous distention of the more upstream colon indicating that this is a relatively chronic process. Attempts at manual disimpaction were unsuccessful. The patient underwent surgical disimpaction, and 20 lb of fecal debris were removed.

DIFFERENTIAL DIAGNOSIS Distal colonic obstruction due to tumor or stricture, delayed diagnosis of Hirschsprung disease.

DIAGNOSIS Delayed diagnosis of Hirschsprung disease.

DISCUSSION Hirschsprung disease (also known as congenital aganglionic megacolon) occurs when neural crest cells fail to migrate appropriately to the distal most part of the rectum. The improperly innervated segment of colon cannot relax properly, which results in a functional obstruction. At barium enema, a transition is seen at the junction of normally innervated but dilated proximal colon and the abnormally innervated, decompressed distal colon.

Usually just the distal most portion of the colon lacks normal innervation, though in less than 10% of cases large portions of the colon or the entire colon may be involved. Men are affected more often than women. Ten percent of patients with Hirschsprung disease also have Down syndrome. Clinically, Hirschsprung disease may be suspected in infancy if the newborn baby does not pass meconium within 48 hours.

Questions for Further Thought

1. What would be the next step to confirm the diagnosis?
2. How is Hirschsprung disease treated?

Reporting Responsibilities

1. Notify the ordering physician that the patient has a distal colonic obstruction which is likely long-standing.
2. Suggest digital rectal examination and/or sigmoidoscopy to rule out a mass such as a rectal cancer as the cause of obstruction.
3. Suggest consideration of rectal biopsy to confirm the diagnosis of Hirschsprung disease.

What the Treating Physician Needs to Know

1. Rectal biopsy is needed to confirm the diagnosis of Hirschsprung disease.

Answers

1. Rectal biopsy. Demonstration of lack of normal ganglion cells would confirm the diagnosis.
2. When diagnosed in infancy, "pull-through" surgery is the usual treatment with the normal segment of colon pulled down and sewn over the abnormal segment of colon. In older patients, the abnormal segment of colon is surgically removed, and the remaining colon is reanastomosed.

REFERENCES

1. Lee NK, Kim S, Jeon TY, et al. Complications of congenital and developmental abnormalities of the gastrointestinal tract in adolescents and adults: evaluation with multimodality imaging. Radiographics 2010;30:1489-1507.
2. Kanne JP, Rohrmann CA Jr, Lichtenstein JE. Eponyms in radiology of the digestive tract: historical perspectives and imaging appearances. Part 1. Pharynx, esophagus, stomach and intestine. Radiographics 2006;26:129-142.

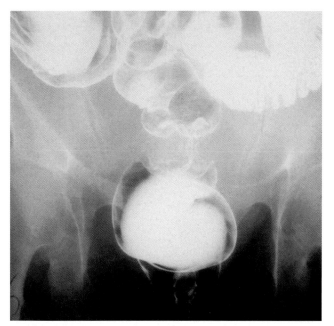

FIGURE 1.43A

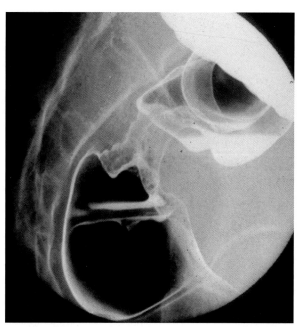

FIGURE 1.43B

FINDINGS Double-contrast barium enema demonstrates circumferential narrowing of the rectosigmoid colon with an "apple core" appearance and mucosal irregularity (A, B).

DIFFERENTIAL DIAGNOSIS Rectal cancer, stricture, endometriosis.

DIAGNOSIS Rectal cancer.

DISCUSSION This lesion is a classic apple core lesion which is highly suspicious for rectal cancer. The mucosal irregularity in this case makes a benign stricture unlikely. Severe endometriosis could have a similar appearance but usually does not result in this degree of luminal narrowing.

Questions for Further Thought

1. What would be the next step to confirm the diagnosis?
2. Name a potential cause of a false-negative barium enema.

Reporting Responsibility

1. Describe the size and location of the constricting mass.

What the Treating Physician Needs to Know

1. This annular constricting rectal mass is highly suspicious for rectal cancer.
2. Colonoscopy with tissue sampling should be performed for further evaluation.

Answers

1. Colonoscopy and biopsy.
2. Small lesions (unlike this case) may be missed if they are obscured by the barium pool.

REFERENCE

1. Levine MS, Rubesin SE, Laufer I, Herlinger H. Diagnosis of colorectal neoplasms at double-contrast barium enema examination. Radiology 2000;216:11-18.

CLINICAL HISTORY *51-year-old woman presents for routine screening double-contrast barium enema.*

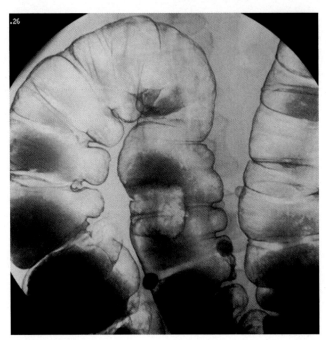

FIGURE 1.44A

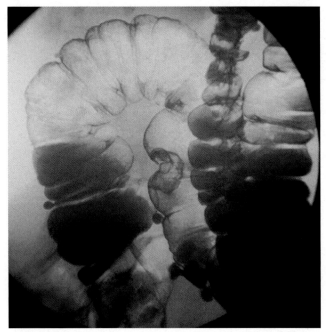

FIGURE 1.44B

FINDINGS An approximately 3.5-cm sessile mass is identified in the proximal transverse colon in barium pool (A) and air-contrast (B) images from a double-contrast barium enema. Scattered colonic diverticula are also noted.

DIFFERENTIAL DIAGNOSIS Colonic adenocarcinoma, polyp, retained stool.

DIAGNOSIS Adenomatous polyp.

DISCUSSION Differential possibilities in this case include a polyp, colonic adenocarcinoma, and retained stool. The fixed position of this mass despite multiple changes in patient positioning and administration of air and barium rules out retained stool. Colonoscopy with biopsy and/or removal of the mass is required to distinguish between a polyp and adenocarcinoma.

Questions for Further Thought

1. What is the relationship between polyp size and malignancy?
2. What are the American Cancer Society's current recommendations for colon cancer screening?

Reporting Responsibilities

1. Describe the size and location of the mass.
2. Describe whether or not the mass is obstructing.

What the Treating Physician Needs to Know

1. The size and location of the mass.
2. If the mass is obstructing.

Answers

1. Risk of cancer increases with polyp size. Risk of cancer for adenomatous polyps <1 cm, 1 to 2 cm, and >2 cm is 1.3%, 9.5%, and 46.0%, respectively, according to Muto et al.
2. American Cancer Society recommendations for colorectal cancer and polyp screening for men and women at average risk beginning at age 50 include flexible sigmoidoscopy every 5 years, or colonoscopy every 10 years, or double-contrast barium enema every 5 years, or CT colonography every 5 years.

REFERENCES

1. Muto T, Bussey HJR, Morson BC. The evolution of cancer of the colon and rectum. Cancer 1975; 36:2251-2270.
2. www.cancer.org. Accessed June 20, 2013.

CLINICAL HISTORY *68-year-old woman undergoing double-contrast barium enema for colon cancer screening.*

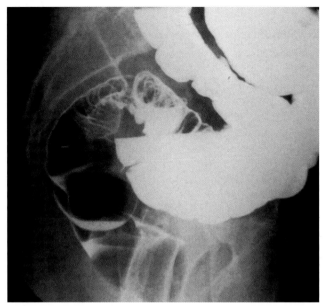

FIGURE 1.45A

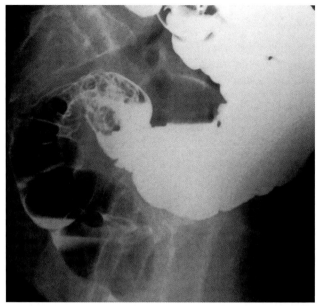

FIGURE 1.45B

FINDINGS Images (A, B) from a double-contrast barium enema demonstrate a focal, approximately 2.5 cm in length area of narrowing of the rectosigmoid colon. The mucosa in this area of narrowing appears mostly smooth.

DIFFERENTIAL DIAGNOSIS Colonic adenocarcinoma, submucosal mass, extrinsic compression (e.g., endometriosis, metastatic disease/carcinomatosis, and adjacent fluid collection).

DIAGNOSIS Extrinsic compression due to endometriosis.

DISCUSSION As with the esophagus and stomach, evaluation of the mucosal surface in an area of narrowing can help distinguish a mucosally based process from a submucosal or extrinsic process. The relatively smooth appearance of the mucosa in the above case therefore favors a submucosal or extrinsic process. CT or MR would be an acceptable next step to evaluate for endometriosis, carcinomatosis, or a pelvic fluid collection resulting in extrinsic compression. Alternatively, colonoscopy may be performed to evaluate the mucosa in this area to exclude a colonic adenocarcinoma. If the abnormality can be identified at colonoscopy, tissue sampling could be performed.

Endometriosis is defined as endometrial tissue abnormally located outside of the uterus. Fewer than 25% of patients with endometriosis have bowel implants. When bowel implants occur, they most commonly involve the rectosigmoid colon followed by the terminal ileum or appendix. Endometrial implants start on the serosal surface but can extend more deeply into the bowel wall.

At double-contrast barium enema, endometrial implants may appear as flattening of the bowel wall, extrinsic impression on the bowel wall, or undulation of the mucosa. In a 2008 study,[1] double-contrast barium enema was found to be 88% sensitive and 93% specific for the diagnosis of pelvic endometriosis. All of these implants measured 2.5 cm or less in this series, and approximately 25% of patients had more than one implant.

Questions for Further Thought

1. What symptoms are associated with endometrial implants along the bowel?
2. How are endometrial implants along the bowel treated?

Reporting Requirements

1. Describe the location of the abnormality.
2. Suggest either CT or MR to look for a soft-tissue mass or fluid collection in the area of narrowing seen on the enema study.
3. Colonoscopy with tissue sampling may also be helpful as described above.

What the Treating Physician Needs to Know

1. This patient has a focal area of colonic narrowing along the rectosigmoid colon.

2. If the endometrial implant is entirely serosal in location, it may not be detectable at colonoscopy. In this scenario, laparoscopy with tissue sampling would be necessary to confirm the diagnosis.

Answers

1. Patients with endometrial implants along the bowel may be asymptomatic or may present with abdominal pain and diarrhea which may be bloody.

2. Endometrial implants isolated to the serosal surface may be shaved off. Endometrial implants that extend more deeply into the bowel wall may require resection of a segment of bowel to remove the implant.

REFERENCE

1. Faccioli N, Manfredi R, Mainardi P, et al. Barium enema evaluation of colonic involvement in endometriosis. Am J Roentgenol 2008;190:1050-1054.

CLINICAL HISTORY *55-year-old woman undergoing double-contrast barium enema for colon cancer screening.*

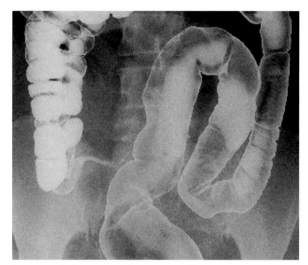

FIGURE 1.46A

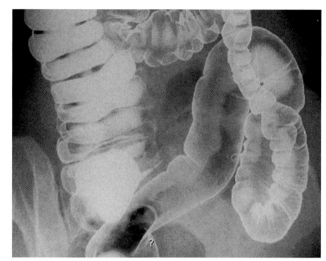

FIGURE 1.46B

FINDINGS Images from a double-contrast barium enema study demonstrate an approximately 6-mm filling defect in the barium pool (A) which is outlined by peripheral contrast material in the air-contrast image (B).

DIFFERENTIAL DIAGNOSIS Diverticulum, fecal debris, polyp.

DIAGNOSIS Polyp.

DISCUSSION At barium enema, a diverticulum will fill with contrast material when it is dependent and will fill with air when it is nondependent. Diverticula usually also protrude beyond the margin of the colon wall. By comparison, a polyp will appear as a filling defect in the barium pool and will be peripherally outlined by contrast material in air-contrast images. The most helpful discriminator for fecal debris is that it is mobile.

Polyps are considered to be precancerous lesions and therefore are usually removed. Small polyps can be removed endoscopically, whereas larger polyps may require surgery.

Question for Further Thought

1. How sensitive is double-contrast barium enema for detection of colonic polyps?

Reporting Requirement

1. Describe the size and location of the colonic polyp. This information will aid the endoscopist who will most likely try to remove this polyp.

What the Treating Physician Needs to Know

1. This patient has a small polyp in the sigmoid colon.

Answer

1. Various numbers are reported in the literature. Sensitivity is dependent on a number of variables including technique and patient preparation. A 2004 study[1] found double-contrast barium enema to be 39% to 56% sensitive for the detection of polyps ≥1 cm. By comparison, a 1989 study[2] found double-contrast barium enema to be 95% sensitive for the detection of polyps ≥1 cm.

REFERENCES

1. Johnson CD, MacCarty RL, Welch TJ, et al. Comparison of the relative sensitivity of CT colonography and double-contrast barium enema for screen detection of colorectal polyps. Clin Gastroenterol Hepatol 2004;2:314-321.
2. Ott DJ, Scharling ED, Chen YM, Wu WC, Gelfand DW. Barium enema examination: sensitivity in detecting colonic polyps and carcinomas. South Med J 1989;82:197-200.

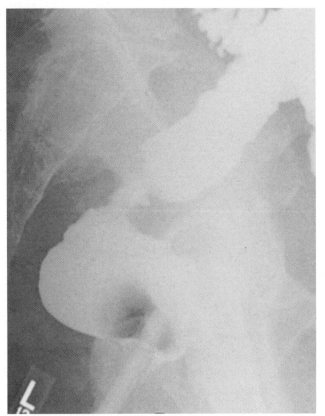

FIGURE 1.47A

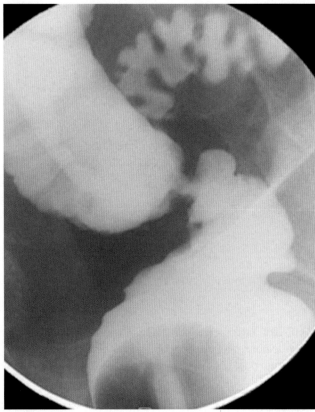

FIGURE 1.47B

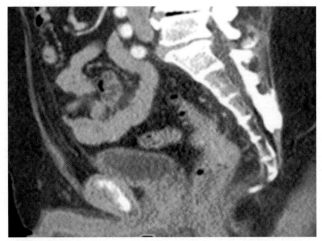

FIGURE 1.47C

DIFFERENTIAL DIAGNOSIS Adenocarcinoma, benign stricture, colitis.

DIAGNOSIS Adenocarcinoma.

DISCUSSION The short-segment nature of the severe narrowing in the above case makes a colitis unlikely. The differential diagnosis is then narrowed to a benign or malignant stricture. The mucosal irregularity is highly suspicious for malignancy. Colonoscopy was performed, and pathology revealed adenocarcinoma.

The CT image is shown to demonstrate how relatively subtle colon cancers can be at routine CT.

Question for Further Thought

1. What is the sensitivity of routine CT for detection of colorectal cancer and large polyps?

Reporting Requirement

1. Describe the location and length of the abnormality as this information will aid the endoscopist in obtaining tissue.

FINDINGS Overhead (A) and spot fluoroscopic image (B) from an enema study demonstrate an approximately 2 cm in length area of focal rectal narrowing with associated mucosal irregularity. Sagittal reformation CT image (C) demonstrates segmental rectal wall thickening corresponding to the area of narrowing seen in the enema study.

What the Treating Physician Needs to Know

1. This patient has a colonic stricture that is highly suspicious for malignancy.
2. Colonoscopy with tissue sampling should be considered to confirm the diagnosis.

Answer

1. A 2010 study[1] found that retrospective segmental review of the colon at routine CT was 65% to 83% sensitive for the detection of colon cancers and 15% sensitive for detection of polyps measuring ≥1 cm.

REFERENCE

1. Ozel B, Pickhardt PJ, Kim DH, Schumacher C, Bhargava N, Winter TC. Accuracy of routine nontargeted CT without colonography technique for the detection of large colorectal polyps and cancer. Dis Colon Rectum 2010;53:911-918.

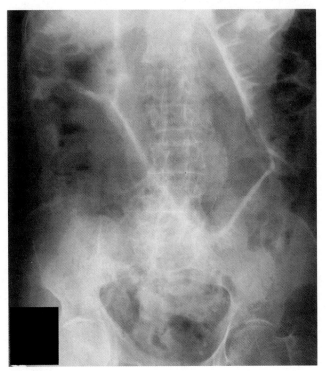

FIGURE 1.48A

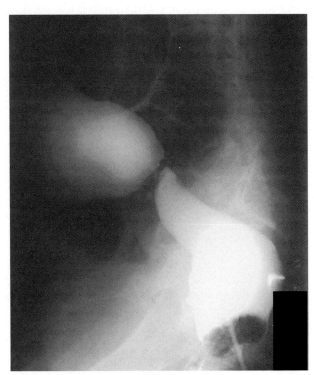

FIGURE 1.48B

FINDINGS Abdominal radiograph (A) demonstrates marked dilation of a loop of bowel extending from the left lower abdomen into the right upper quadrant. Note also distention of the imaged right colon and left colon. The transverse colon was also distended (not shown). Water-soluble enema study (B) demonstrates an abrupt narrowing of the sigmoid colon with a "bird-beak" appearance.

DIFFERENTIAL DIAGNOSIS BASED ON INITIAL RADIO-GRAPH Cecal volvulus, colonic ileus, distal colonic obstruction, sigmoid volvulus.

DIAGNOSIS Sigmoid volvulus.

DISCUSSION Sigmoid volvulus occurs when the sigmoid colon twists on itself, usually resulting in a closed-loop bowel obstruction. The dilated closed-loop segment of the obstructed sigmoid colon can become markedly dilated and usually extends out of the pelvis into the right upper quadrant or left upper quadrant. The opposing walls of dilated sigmoid colon appear as a white line simulating the crease of a coffee bean, a finding termed the "coffee bean sign."

When markedly dilated colon is visible at radiography, the differential diagnosis also includes cecal volvulus, a severe ileus, or a distal colonic obstruction due to causes other than volvulus. A helpful clue to distinguish cecal volvulus from sigmoid volvulus is the amount of dilated upstream colon. In the setting of sigmoid volvulus, the upstream colon (ascending, transverse, and descending) is usually distended. By comparison, in the setting of cecal volvulus, the majority of the colon (ascending, transverse, and descending) is usually relatively decompressed as it is downstream from the site of volvulus.

It can sometimes be difficult to distinguish a severe colonic ileus or colonic obstruction due to other etiologies from a sigmoid volvulus. For example, bed-bound patients with chronic narcotic use may present with a massively dilated colon due to a severe ileus that can simulate sigmoid volvulus at radiography. Therefore, water-soluble enema study is often performed in suspected cases of volvulus to confirm the diagnosis. The enema will demonstrate an abrupt narrowing of the contrast column at the site of the twist which has a "bird-beak" appearance. Contrast material may or may not reach beyond the site of the twist.

The diagnosis of sigmoid volvulus also can be made at CT. Administering rectal contrast material can be helpful in making the CT diagnosis. CT imaging findings of sigmoid volvulus are swirling mesenteric vessels at the site of volvulus, marked dilation of the sigmoid colon, distention of the colon upstream from the twist, and tapering of the rectal contrast material column at the level of the twist.

Questions for Further Thought

1. Is cecal volvulus or sigmoid volvulus more common?
2. How is sigmoid volvulus managed?

Reporting Requirements

1. Based on the initial film, report that findings are suspicious for sigmoid volvulus.
2. Suggest a water-soluble enema study for confirmation.

What the Treating Physician Needs to Know

1. The enema findings are diagnostic of sigmoid volvulus.
2. Gastroenterology or surgical consultation should be considered for volvulus reduction.

Answers

1. Sigmoid volvulus is much more common than cecal volvulus and accounts for up to 75% of cases of colonic volvulus in some series.
2. Sigmoid volvulus requires urgent reduction due to the risk of bowel ischemia and infarction if left untreated. Sigmoidoscopy may be used to reduce the volvulus; however, up to 90% of patients will experience a recurrence. Surgical fixation of or resection of the sigmoid colon is considered definitive treatment.

REFERENCES

1. Peterson CM, Anderson JS, Hara AK, Carenza JW, Menias CO. Volvulus of the gastrointestinal tract: appearances at multimodality imaging. Radiographics 2009;29:1281-1293.
2. Feldman D. The coffee bean sign. Radiology 2000;216:178-179.

CLINICAL HISTORY *56-year-old man with rectal bleeding.*

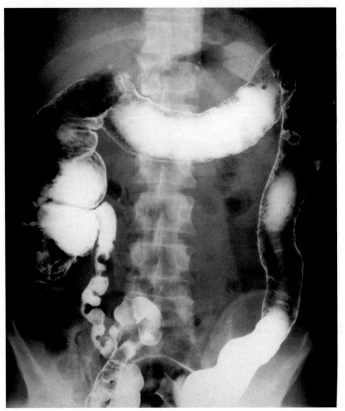

FIGURE 1.49A

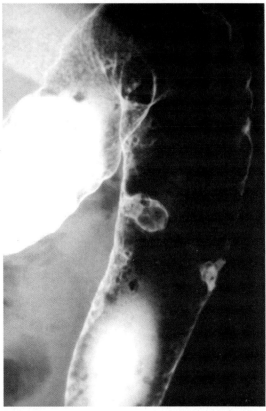

FIGURE 1.49B

FINDINGS Overhead image (A) from a double-contrast barium enema demonstrates loss of the usual colonic haustral fold pattern, most pronounced from the transverse colon through the imaged sigmoid colon. Note several polypoid structures in the left colon. Magnified image (B) demonstrates two dominant polypoid structures coated with barium in the splenic flexure of the colon.

DIFFERENTIAL DIAGNOSIS Adenomatous polyps, pseudopolyps due to ulcerative colitis.

DIAGNOSIS Pseudopolyps due to ulcerative colitis.

DISCUSSION Loss of the usual colonic haustral fold pattern in the above case is indicative of long-standing ulcerative colitis. This appearance of the colon is referred to as "lead pipe colon" and is thought to reflect hypertrophy of the muscularis mucosa and deposition of fibrous tissue in the colonic wall.

Ulcerative colitis is a superficial mucosal process that begins in the rectum and extends proximally. The inflamed mucosal surface of the colon ulcerates and sloughs off. Confluent areas of sloughed mucosa are common. Residual patches of normal mucosa appear as pseudopolyps as in the above case.

Ulcerative colitis is a form of inflammatory bowel disease and is thought to result from a combination of genetic and environmental factors. Most patients with this condition are diagnosed as teenagers or young adults and present with diarrhea, weight loss, and fever. Treatment is usually medical management with total colectomy performed for those with medically refractory disease. Individuals with ulcerative colitis are at increased risk for colonic adenocarcinoma.

Question for Further Thought

1. What is toxic megacolon?

Reporting Requirement

1. Describe the presence of lead pipe colon and pseudopolyps reflecting sequelae of ulcerative colitis.

What the Treating Physician Needs to Know

1. If there is evidence of colonic obstruction as ulcerative colitis patients may develop colonic strictures.
2. If there is evidence of adenocarcinoma given the increased risk of colonic adenocarcinoma in individuals with ulcerative colitis.

Answer

1. Toxic megacolon is characterized by colonic dilatation to >6 cm in diameter and systemic toxicity. Approximately 5% of patients with ulcerative colitis develop toxic megacolon that can be fatal.

REFERENCES

1. Roggeveen MJ, Tismenetsky M, Shapiro R. Ulcerative colitis. Radiographics 2006;26:947-951.
2. Horton KM, Corl FM, Fishman EK. CT evaluation of the colon: inflammatory disease. Radiographics 2000;20:399-418.

CASE 1.50

CLINICAL HISTORY *33-year-old man with a family history of colon cancer.*

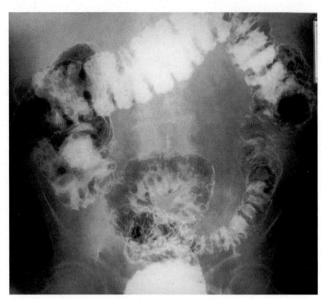

FIGURE 1.50

FINDINGS Double-contrast barium enema demonstrates innumerable polypoid filling defects in the patient's colon.

DIFFERENTIAL DIAGNOSIS Numerous sporadic polyps, FAP.

DIAGNOSIS FAP.

DISCUSSION The very large number of polyps in this case and the relatively young age of the patient favors FAP. FAP is an autosomal dominant genetic disorder characterized by the development of hundreds to thousands of colonic polyps. The risk of colon cancer is nearly 100% in patients with FAP, and a majority of patients will develop a colon cancer by age 39 if left untreated. Therefore, these patients routinely undergo colectomy. The average age at onset of polyposis is 16. While colon cancer is the most common malignancy in these patients, adenocarcinoma of the duodenum and papilla of Vater is the second most common malignancy. Patients with FAP may also develop desmoid tumors.

Questions for Further Thought

1. What would be the next step to confirm the diagnosis?
2. Name two syndromes associated with FAP.

Reporting Responsibility

1. Describe the numerous polyps and suggest the possibility of FAP.

What the Treating Physician Needs to Know

1. A patient with FAP will most likely develop colon cancer if the patient does not undergo colectomy.
2. In addition to the syndromes described below, patients with FAP are also at increased risk for thyroid cancer and hepatoblastoma.

Answers

1. Genetic testing for a mutation in the adenomatous polyposis coli (*APC*) gene is performed to make the diagnosis of FAP.
2. Gardner syndrome (osteomas, dental abnormalities, soft-tissue tumors such as epidermoid cysts, fibromas, and desmoid tumors) and Turcot syndrome (medulloblastoma) are both associated with FAP.

REFERENCES

1. Galiatsatos P, Foulkes WD. Familial adenomatous polyposis. Am J Gastroenterol 2006;101:385-398.
2. Hughes MR, Huang EH. Molecular basis of hereditary colon cancer. Sem Col Rect Surg 2011;22:65-70.

CLINICAL HISTORY *58-year-old man with abdominal pain.*

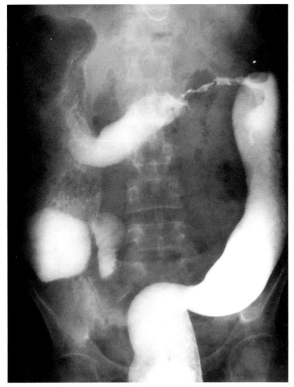

FIGURE 1.51A

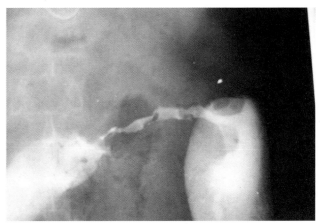

FIGURE 1.51B

FINDINGS Overhead image (A) and magnified image (B) from an enema study demonstrate an approximately 8 cm in length area of mucosal irregularity and luminal narrowing involving the distal transverse colon. Note also the loss of the expected colonic haustral fold pattern that gives the colon a "lead pipe" appearance.

DIFFERENTIAL DIAGNOSIS Adenocarcinoma, benign stricture.

DIAGNOSIS Adenocarcinoma in the setting of ulcerative colitis.

DISCUSSION The stricture in the above case is a colon cancer until proven otherwise. The above patient underwent colonoscopy, and a diagnosis of colonic adenocarcinoma was established. The loss of the usual colonic haustral pattern in this case with a "lead pipe colon" appearance is indicative of long-standing ulcerative colitis.

Patients with ulcerative colitis have an increased risk of colonic adenocarcinoma when compared with the general population. Ulcerative colitis patients have an approximately 20% risk of developing colonic adenocarcinoma within 30 years after the diagnosis of ulcerative colitis.

Ulcerative colitis is a form of inflammatory bowel disease that is thought to result from a combination of environmental and genetic factors. Patients are usually diagnosed with ulcerative colitis between the ages of 15 and 30 after presenting with recurrent episodes of diarrhea, fever, and abdominal pain.

Ulcerative colitis primarily affects the mucosal layer of the colon with disease involvement usually beginning at the anus and progressing proximally in a contiguous fashion. Over time, involved portions of the colon may develop a "lead pipe" appearance due to deposition of fibrous tissue in the bowel wall and muscular hypertrophy. Ulcerative colitis may also be complicated by colonic strictures and adenocarcinoma as in the above case. Fewer than 10% of patients with ulcerative colitis also develop primary sclerosing cholangitis.

Crohn disease is also a common form of inflammatory bowel disease that, like, ulcerative colitis is usually diagnosed in older teenagers and young adults. However, the pattern of bowel involvement is quite different in Crohn disease when compared with ulcerative colitis. For example, Crohn disease is characterized by transmural involvement of the GI tract with skip lesions. The terminal ileum is the most common site of involvement, though Crohn disease can impact any part of the GI tract from the esophagus to the anus. Given its transmural nature, Crohn disease may be complicated by fistulas and abscess formation. Individuals with Crohn disease may also develop fibrostenotic strictures.

REFERENCES

1. Eaden JA, Abrams KR, Mayberry JF. The risk of colorectal cancer in ulcerative colitis: a meta-analysis. Gut 2001;48:526-535.
2. Olsson R, Danielsson A, Jarnerot G, et al. Prevalence of primary sclerosing cholangitis in patients with ulcerative colitis. Gastroenterol 1991;100:1319-1323.

CHAPTER 2

Computed Tomography (CT) Imaging

CLINICAL HISTORY *34-year-old man with fever and abdominal pain.*

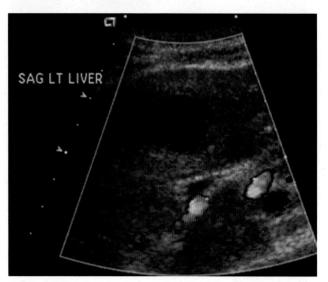

FIGURE 2.1A

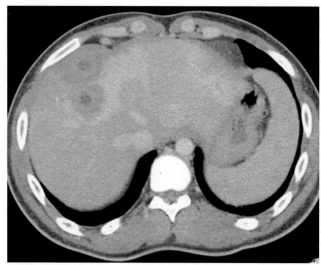

FIGURE 2.1B

FINDINGS Color Doppler ultrasound (US) (A) demonstrates a 3-cm hypoechoic mass in the left hepatic lobe without definite internal blood flow. Multiple other similar lesions were seen at US. Contrast-enhanced computed tomography (CT) (B) demonstrates multiple low-attenuation hepatic lesions with central cystic spaces and surrounding areas of relative hyperenhancement.

DIFFERENTIAL DIAGNOSIS Abscesses, cysts, cystic metastases.

DIAGNOSIS Abscesses.

DISCUSSION The "double-target" sign seen in the above case refers to the cystic central portion of an abscess surrounded by reactive hyperemia. At T1-weighted magnetic resonance (MR), abscesses usually demonstrate dark signal. At T2-weighted MR, perilesional edema may be seen but can also be seen with liver metastases. Abscesses may also appear as a large, multilocular area of low attenuation.

Cystic metastases can occur when hypervascular masses outgrow their blood supply and become necrotic. Treated gastrointestinal stromal tumor (GIST) metastases, for example, can have a cystic appearance. Clinical correlation can help distinguish between liver abscesses and metastases, but percutaneous biopsy is sometimes needed. Cysts appear entirely cystic at CT or MR and do not demonstrate adjacent reactive hyperemia.

Questions for Further Thought

1. What are the most common organisms found in liver abscesses?
2. By what route(s) do bacteria enter the liver?

Reporting Requirements

1. Describe the size, number, and location of liver lesions.
2. Include hepatic abscess in the differential diagnosis of a cystic liver mass with surrounding hyperemia.

What the Treating Physician Needs to Know

1. For larger abscesses, image-guided percutaneous drainage catheter placement may be beneficial.
2. Up to 26% of patients may become septic (fever, hypotension, rigors, and hypoxia) immediately following percutaneous drainage catheter placement even in the setting of prophylactic antibiotics.

Answers

1. *Escherichia coli*, *Clostridium*, and *Bacteroides* are the most common species found in liver abscesses.
2. Bacteria enter the liver most frequently via the portal system or the biliary system.

REFERENCES

1. Mortele KJ, Ros PR. Cystic focal liver lesions in the adult: differential CT and MR imaging features. Radiographics 2001;21:895-910.
2. Thomas J, Turner SR, Nelson RC, Paulson EK. Postprocedure sepsis in imaging-guided percutaneous hepatic abscess drainage: how often does it occur? Am J Roentgenol 2006;186:1419-1422.

CLINICAL HISTORY *Three different patients with vague abdominal discomfort.*

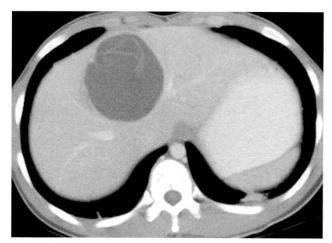

FIGURE 2.2A

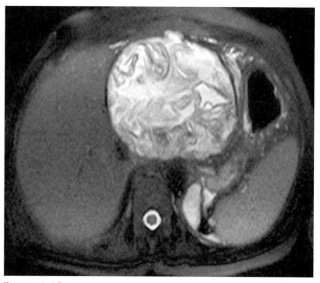

FIGURE 2.2B

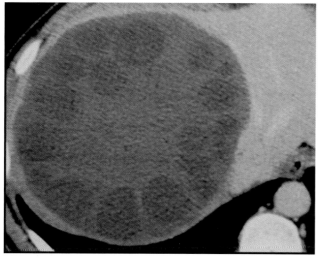

FIGURE 2.2C

FINDINGS Contrast-enhanced CT (A) demonstrates a 10-cm low-attenuation mass spanning the right and left hepatic lobes. Linear areas of increased attenuation are visible in the nondependent portion of the mass. A small, geographic area of low attenuation is seen along the right aspect of the mass most likely reflecting some adjacent edema.

T2-weighted MR in a different patient (B) demonstrates a 12-cm left hepatic lobe lesion which is T2 bright and contains numerous curvilinear low signal areas. Contrast-enhanced CT in a third patient (C) demonstrates a 15-cm right hepatic lobe mass with several round structures internally.

DIFFERENTIAL DIAGNOSIS Bacterial abscesses, biliary cystadenomas, hydatid cysts.

DIAGNOSIS Hydatid cysts.

DISCUSSION Hydatid disease is caused by Echinococcus granulosus and is endemic in many parts of the world, including the Middle East, the Mediterranean, and South America. At histology, the margin of the cyst is termed the "pericyst" and is composed of compressed liver parenchyma and inflammatory cells. The cyst wall contains an outer acellular layer (ectocyst) and an inner germinal membrane (endocyst).

When all three layers (pericyst, ectocyst, and endocyst) are adherent to one another, the hydatid cyst will appear as a unilocular cystic structure that cannot be distinguished from a simple cyst. When the inner ectocyst and endocyst become detached from the pericyst, they will float within the cyst giving rise to the "water lily sign" (A, B). An additional characteristic pattern of hydatid cyst disease seen at imaging is the daughter cyst appearance where numerous smaller cystic structures are seen within a dominant cyst as in (C) above.

Bacterial abscesses are usually less well defined than the above lesions. Also, bacterial abscesses may be multiloculated and have a lobulated rather than a spherical margin. Bacterial abscesses may contain internal enhancing septations.

Biliary cystadenomas are often well circumscribed, but are usually not as spherical as the above mass. Biliary cystadenomas usually have internal septations and often have an enhancing soft tissue component.

Question for Further Thought

1. What other organs can be affected by hydatid disease?

Reporting Responsibilities

1. Describe the size and location of the lesion and whether or not there is mass effect on adjacent structures.
2. If a water lily sign or daughter cyst sign is seen, it is highly likely that the lesion is a hydatid cyst.

What the Treating Physician Needs to Know

1. The water lily sign and the daughter cyst sign are highly specific for hydatid disease.
2. Hydatid cysts are usually resected.

3. Many hydatid cysts appear as unilocular cystic structures that cannot be distinguished from simple cysts.

Answer

1. Hydatid cysts may be seen in almost any location in the body, including the lungs, brain, spleen, and kidneys.

REFERENCES

1. Acunas B, Rozanes I, Acunas G, Celik L, Alper A, Gokmen E. Hydatid cyst of the liver: identification of detached cyst lining on CT scans obtained after cyst puncture. Am J Roentgenol 1992;156:751-753.
2. Pedrosa I, Saiz A, Arrazola J, Ferreiros J, Pedrosa CS. Hydatid disease: radiologic and pathologic features and complications. Radiographics 2000;20:795-817.

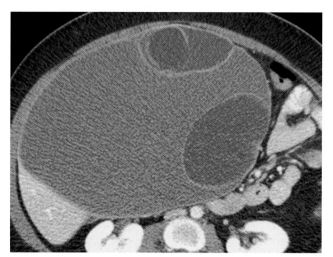

FIGURE 2.3A

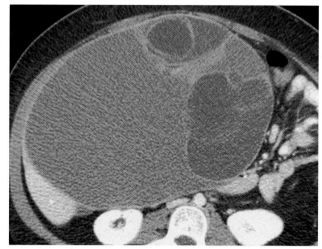

FIGURE 2.3B

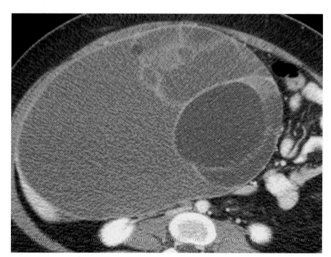

FIGURE 2.3C

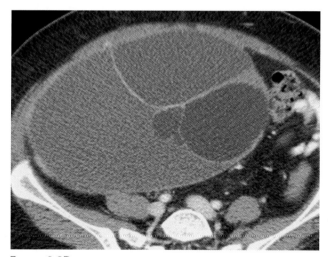

FIGURE 2.3D

FINDINGS Contrast-enhanced CT demonstrates a 20-cm mass involving the left and right hepatic lobes. Multiple enhancing internal septations are seen (A-D) as well as areas of soft tissue enhancement (B,C).

DIFFERENTIAL DIAGNOSIS Abscess, biliary cystadenoma, biliary cystadenocarcinoma.

DIAGNOSIS Biliary cystadenoma.

DISCUSSION Biliary cystadenomas are uncommon cystic liver masses. These lesions most commonly occur in middle-aged women who may present with vague abdominal discomfort due to mass effect from the lesion. The etiology of biliary cystadenomas is unknown, but a congenital origin due to aberrant development of a biliary anlage has been proposed.

At CT, biliary cystadenomas appear as multilocular cystic masses that contain internal enhancing septations, mural nodules, and occasionally calcifications. The presence of a solid enhancing component does not necessarily indicate malignancy. Cystadenomas can therefore be difficult to distinguish from cystadenocarcinomas at imaging. These lesions usually demonstrate bright signal at T2-weighted MR. T1 signal intensity varies depending on the protein content of the cyst fluid.

Histologically, biliary cystadenomas usually appear as multilocular cystic masses lined by a cuboidal or columnar epithelium that resembles biliary epithelium. A majority of cystadenomas also contain ovarian stroma.

Biliary cystadenomas can be distinguished from simple cysts based on the presence of internal enhancing septations and enhancing soft tissue. Abscesses are usually less well defined, do not demonstrate enhancing solid nodules, and may demonstrate adjacent edema. Biliary cystadenomas can be difficult to distinguish from biliary cystadenocarcinomas. Biliary cystadenomas are usually resected due to the risk of malignant transformation and the difficulty in completely excluding cystadenocarcinoma at imaging.

Questions for Further Thought

1. In what other locations may biliary cystadenomas occur?
2. What imaging features distinguish biliary cystadenoma from biliary cystadenocarcinoma?

Reporting Responsibilities

1. Report the size and location of the lesion.
2. Report the relationship of the lesion to major vascular structures as this information may impact surgical planning.

What the Treating Physician Needs to Know

1. Biliary cystadenomas are usually surgical lesions and are resected due to the risk of malignant transformation.

2. Biliary cystadenomas cannot be reliably differentiated from biliary cystadenocarcinomas at imaging.

Answers

1. Biliary cystadenomas also may occur in the gallbladder or in the extrahepatic biliary system. The majority of biliary cystadenomas occur in the liver.
2. Unfortunately, no imaging features reliably distinguish biliary cystadenoma from biliary cystadenocarcinoma. Both are surgical lesions.

REFERENCES

1. Mortele KJ, Ros PR. Cystic focal liver lesions in the adult: differential CT and MR imaging features. Radiographics 2001;21:895-910.
2. Horton KM, Bluemke DA, Hruban RH, Soyer P, Fishman EK. CT and MR imaging of benign hepatic and biliary tumors. Radiographics 1999;19:431-451.
3. Levy AD, Murakata LA, Abbott RM, Rohrmann Jr CA. From the archives of the AFIP: benign tumors and tumor-like lesions of the gallbladder and extrahepatic bile ducts: radiologic-pathologic correlation. Radiographics 2002;22:387-413.

CLINICAL HISTORY *68-year-old man with lung cancer, restaging examination.*

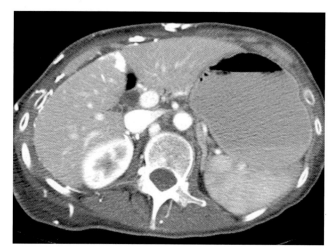

FIGURE 2.4A

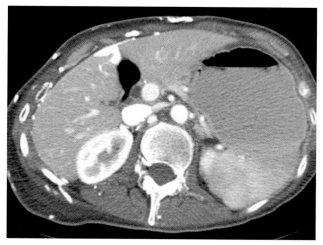

FIGURE 2.4B

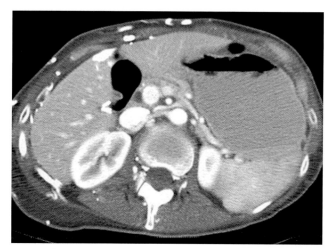

FIGURE 2.4C

FINDINGS Contrast enhanced CT (A-C) demonstrates an avidly enhancing triangular-shaped area in the periphery of the segment 4 liver. Note also numerous collateral vessels in the subcutaneous tissues.

DIFFERENTIAL DIAGNOSIS Hypervascular metastasis, superior vena cava (SVC) occlusion.

DIAGNOSIS SVC occlusion.

DISCUSSION The triangular shape and characteristic enhancement pattern in the segment 4 liver seen in this case is an "Aunt Minnie" for SVC occlusion. Chest CT should be recommended to evaluate for a thoracic mass resulting in SVC occlusion.

The segment 4 liver hyperenhances in the setting of SVC occlusion because of the shunting of large volumes of blood through this area via a portosystemic collateral pathway that develops between subcutaneous collateral vessels and the left portal vein via the paraumbilical vein. Blood passes through the portal vein, liver, hepatic veins, and inferior vena cava (IVC) and returns to the heart via this alternate route.

Patients with SVC occlusion may present with distended neck veins, headache, head and neck swelling, and dyspnea. At ^{99m}Tc-sulfur colloid imaging, patients with SVC occlusion may demonstrate focal accumulation of radiotracer in the segment 4 liver known as the "hot quadrate sign." The quadrate lobe is the segment 4 liver.

Questions for Further Thought

1. What are the most common etiologies of SVC occlusion?
2. Name another collateral pathway in patients with SVC occlusion.

Reporting Responsibilities

1. Report that findings most likely reflect SVC occlusion.
2. Recommend chest CT to evaluate for an obstructing mass.

What the Treating Physician Needs to Know

1. The patient most likely has an occluded SVC.
2. A chest CT is needed to evaluate for a neoplasm occluding the SVC.

Answers

1. Malignancy (e.g., lung cancer) and chronic occlusion due to scarring from multiple central venous access catheters are the most common etiologies of SVC occlusion.

2. The azygous/hemiazygous and paravertebral system is another collateral pathway via which blood can return to the heart in patients with SVC occlusion.

REFERENCES

1. Sheth S, Ebert MD, Fishman EK. Superior vena cava obstruction: evaluation with MDCT. Am J Roentgenol 2010;194:W336-W346.

2. Dickson AM. The focal hepatic hot spot sign. Radiology 2005;237:647-648.

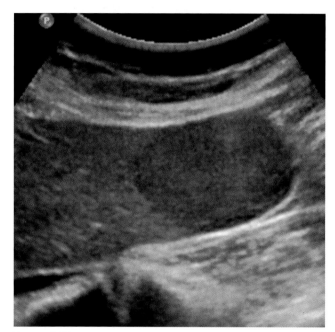

FIGURE 2.5A

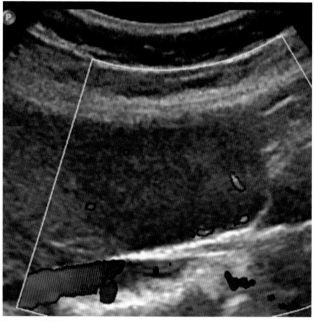

FIGURE 2.5B

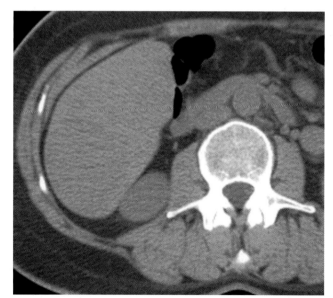

FIGURE 2.5C

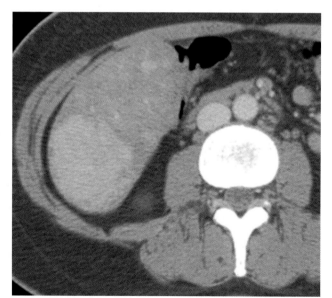

FIGURE 2.5D

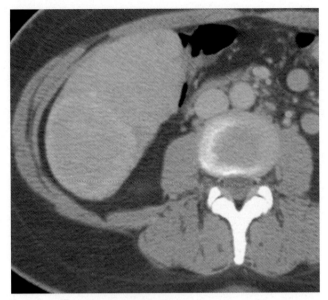

FIGURE 2.5E

FINDINGS Grayscale US (A) demonstrates a 6-cm homogeneous hypoechoic mass in the inferior right hepatic lobe. Blood flow is visible in the mass at color Doppler imaging (B). Patient also underwent CT, and the lesion was low-attenuation precontrast (A), hyperenhanced in the arterial phase (B), and remained more attenuating than the surrounding liver at venous phase imaging (C). An additional smaller, 1.5-cm lesion is visible slightly more anteriorly in the arterial phase image (B).

DIFFERENTIAL DIAGNOSIS Focal nodular hyperplasia (FNH), hepatocellular adenoma, hepatocellular cancer.

DIAGNOSIS Hepatocellular adenoma.

DISCUSSION Hepatocellular adenomas are hyperenhancing lesions that most often occur in women taking oral contraceptive pills, in individuals with glycogen storage disease, and in individuals using anabolic steroids.

Histologically, adenomas appear as sheets of relatively normal-appearing hepatocytes with intervening sinusoids and relatively little connective tissue. Blood supply is via peripheral arterial vessels. The paucity of supporting connective tissue and the presence of arterial pressure blood flow are thought to be factors predisposing these lesions to bleeding. Adenomas do not contain bile ducts, a feature that distinguishes them from areas of FNH at histology.

The US appearance of adenomas is nonspecific. Adenomas may appear hypoechoic (as in this case) or hyperechoic due to the presence of internal blood products.

Adenomas may also have a variable appearance at CT. If the adenoma has bled, it will appear heterogeneous at precontrast CT with areas of low and high precontrast attenuation. The adenoma in this case had not bled and appeared homogeneous at noncontrast CT. Adenomas characteristically hyperenhance in the arterial phase of imaging as compared with the neighboring liver parenchyma. Adenomas are also typically visible in the portal venous phase of enhancement though the amount of enhancement relative to the adjacent liver parenchyma is variable.

At MR, signal loss may be visible at out-of-phase imaging due to intracellular fat. At MR, adenomas are typically bright at T2 though not fluid bright like hemangiomas. T1 signal varies and may be dark or, if blood products are present, bright T1 signal may be visible. As with CT, adenomas hyperenhance in the arterial phase at MR and remain visible in the portal venous phase.

By comparison, FNH appears "stealth" in precontrast images and is often imperceptible or only faintly perceptible. Like adenomas, FNHs hyperenhance in the arterial phase. FNHs are also usually relatively stealth in the portal venous phase. Unlike adenomas, FNHs do not contain fat and therefore do not lose signal at out-of-phase MR.

Adenomas may be difficult to distinguish from hepatocellular cancer as both hyperenhance in the arterial phase and both may contain fat. Hepatocellular cancer usually demonstrates washout at delayed-phase imaging (e.g., 3 minutes post contrast). Adenomas may also demonstrate relative washout. Clinical history, evaluation of the background liver, and correlation with serum α-fetoprotein (AFP) may help distinguish between hepatocellular adenoma and hepatocellular cancer. For example, hepatocellular cancers most commonly occur in patients with chronic liver disease (e.g., small nodular livers), whereas hepatocellular adenomas often occur in patients with morphologically normal livers. AFP may be elevated in the setting of hepatocellular cancer but is usually not elevated in the setting of hepatocellular adenoma.

Questions for Further Thought

1. What is the usual management of hepatocellular adenomas?
2. How does the management of adenomas vary from the management of FNH?

Reporting Requirements

1. Report the size and location of the lesion.
2. Attempt to narrow differential diagnosis as much as possible.

What the Treating Physician Needs to Know

1. Solitary hepatocellular adenomas may be resected due to the risk of bleeding and malignant transformation. Risk of bleeding correlates with adenoma size. The surgical literature suggests that adenomas <5 cm should be followed

with imaging to assess for interval growth. Adenomas >5 cm should be resected, given the potential for bleeding and malignant transformation. However, some surgeons will also resect adenomas that measure smaller than 5 cm in size.

2. Patients with multiple adenomas may undergo embolization procedures and/or resection.

Answers

1. Depending on patient comorbidities and lesion size, adenomas may be resected due to the risk of bleeding and potential for malignant transformation. Patients with multiple adenomas for which resection of all lesions are not possible may undergo embolization. Alternatively,

follow-up imaging following cessation of oral contraceptive pills or anabolic steroids may be recommended to evaluate whether an adenoma regresses.

2. Unlike adenomas for which treatment is often offered, patients with FNH usually require no further treatment. Therefore, management decisions will change depending on whether a lesion is favored to be an adenoma or FNH at imaging.

REFERENCES

1. Faria SC, Iyer RB, Rashid A, Whitman GJ. Hepatic adenoma. Am J Roentgenol 2004;182:1520.
2. Grazioli L, Federle MP, Brancatelli G, Ichikawa T, Olivetti L, Blachar A. Hepatic adenomas: imaging and pathologic findings. Radiographics 2001;21:877-894.

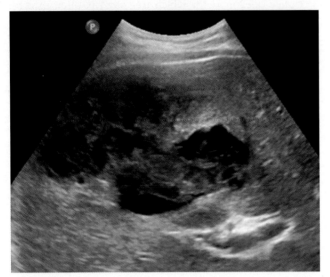

FIGURE 2.6A

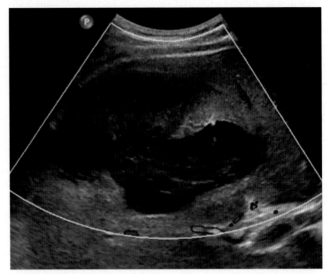

FIGURE 2.6B

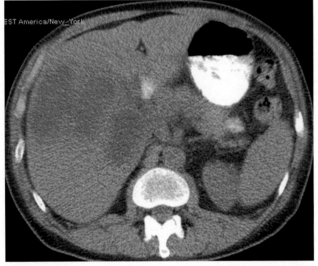

FIGURE 2.6C

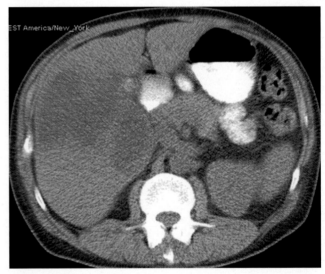

FIGURE 2.6D

FINDINGS Grayscale US (A) demonstrates a 12-cm bilobed, heterogeneous structure in the right hepatic lobe extending toward the liver dome. No definite internal blood flow is seen in this location at color Doppler imaging (B). Mobile debris was visible at real-time imaging. Noncontrast CT (C, D) demonstrates the lesion to be multilobular and of low attenuation.

DIFFERENTIAL DIAGNOSIS Abscess, biloma, hematoma.

DIAGNOSIS Abscess.

DISCUSSION US demonstrates a large structure with internal debris and no internal blood flow. Based on US alone, the structure could be a large abscess, biloma, or hematoma. Given the low attenuation seen at noncontrast CT, a hematoma is unlikely. Blood products at noncontrast CT of the abdomen usually measure >40 to 50 HU. Attenuation values may be lower if blood mixes with ascitic fluid, in anemic patients, and over time as blood products evolve. Given that the low-attenuation areas in the above liver measure approximately 25 HU, a hematoma is unlikely. Bilomas are usually <20 HU attenuation and appear closer to the attenuation of water than hematomas.

Based on imaging features, abscess is the most likely diagnosis in this case. Clinical history of fever and elevated white blood cell count were confirmatory.

Questions for Further Thought

1. What are the most common causes of liver abscesses?
2. The treating physician asks you to drain this abscess. What is your response?

Reporting Requirements

1. Describe the size and location of the abscess.
2. Report should be called to the ordering physician as, if left untreated, mortality is high in patients with liver abscesses.

What the Treating Physician Needs to Know

1. The above lesion is compatible with an abscess.
2. The above lesion would be amenable to percutaneous drainage.

Answers

1. Biliary infections or gastrointestinal (GI) infections drained through the portal venous system are the most common causes of liver abscesses. Therefore, in patients with liver abscesses the biliary system should be evaluated for evidence of obstructing stone, stricture, or tumor. The GI tract should also be evaluated for infection such as appendicitis or diverticulitis.

2. This abscess would be amenable to percutaneous drainage using CT or US guidance. As patients with liver abscesses are prone to sepsis following manipulation of the abscess, it is important to confirm that the patient has received antibiotics prior to the drainage procedure. Aspirated fluid should be sent for culture.

REFERENCES

1. Mortele KJ, Ros PR. Cystic focal liver lesions in the adult: differential CT and MR imaging features. Radiographics 2001;21:895-910.
2. Thomas J, Turner SR, Nelson RC, Paulson EK. Postprocedure sepsis in imaging-guided percutaneous hepatic abscess drainage: how often does it occur? Am J Roentgenol 2006;186:1419-1422.

CLINICAL HISTORY *53-year-old man with hepatitis C undergoing screening for hepatocellular cancer.*

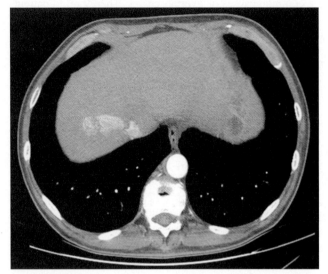

FIGURE 2.7A

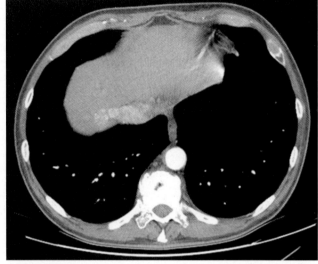

FIGURE 2.7B

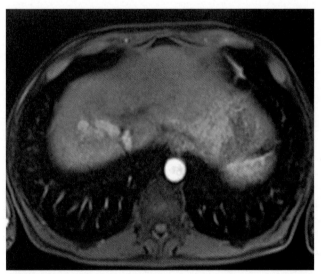

FIGURE 2.7C

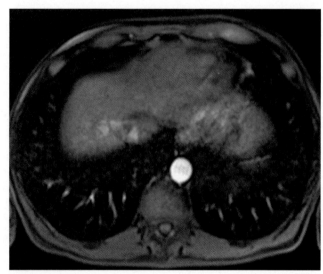

FIGURE 2.7D

FINDINGS Arterial phase contrast-enhanced CT (A) and MR (C) demonstrate a 2-cm round arterially enhancing structure adjacent to the right hepatic vein. The right hepatic vein is expanded by hyperenhancing material that also extends into the IVC (B, D).

DIFFERENTIAL DIAGNOSIS Hepatocellular cancer with associated bland thrombus, hepatocellular cancer with associated tumor thrombus

DIAGNOSIS Hepatocellular cancer with tumor thrombus in the right hepatic vein extending into the IVC.

DISCUSSION Specific diagnostic criteria for hepatocellular carcinoma (HCC) at CT or MR are arterial hyperenhancement (as above) with washout at delayed-phase imaging with a capsule or pseudocapsule (not shown , please see cases in MR chapter).

Treatment options for HCC include resection, liver transplant, and chemoembolization. Patients with small tumors and an otherwise normal or near-normal liver may undergo resection. Patients with unresectable hepatocellular cancers that fall within Milan criteria are candidates for liver transplant. Milan criteria are not more than three tumors ≤3 cm or one tumor ≤5 cm. Based on the 2 cm size of the above tumor, the patient would have been within Milan criteria. However, the presence of tumor thrombus in the IVC or the portal vein currently is considered a contraindication to liver transplant, so the above patient was not a transplant candidate.

Bland thrombus (usually in the portal vein) can also occur in patients with chronic liver disease and portal hypertension. As bland thrombus is not necessarily a contraindication for liver transplant, it is critically important to accurately distinguish between bland thrombus and tumor thrombus. A key feature that distinguishes tumor thrombus from bland thrombus is enhancement of the tumor thrombus. By comparison, bland thrombus does not enhance. Note in the above case the expansion of the right hepatic vein with hyperenhancing material. Neither the middle hepatic vein nor the left hepatic vein is similarly hyperenhancing.

Question for Further Thought

1. In addition to hepatocellular cancer, what other abdominal tumors may directly extend into major vascular structures.

Reporting Requirements

1. Report the size and location of the hepatocellular cancer.
2. Report the presence of tumor thrombus extending into the hepatic vein and IVC.

What the Treating Physician Needs to Know

1. This patient has a hepatocellular cancer with tumor thrombus filling the right hepatic vein and extending into the IVC.

Answer

1. Renal cell cancers may extend into the renal vein and IVC. Adrenal cortical carcinomas may extend into the IVC.

REFERENCES

1. Mazzaferro V, Regalia E, Doci R, et al. Liver transplantation for treatment of small hepatocellular carcinomas in patients with cirrhosis. N Engl J Med 1996;334:693-700.
2. Wald C, Russo MW, Heimbach JK, Hussain HK, Pomfret EA, Bruix J. New OPTN/UNOS policy for liver transplant allocation: standardization of liver imaging, diagnosis, classification and reporting of hepatocellular cancer. Radiology 2013;266:376-382.

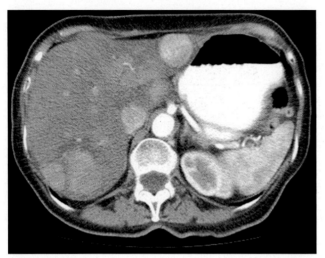

FIGURE 2.8A

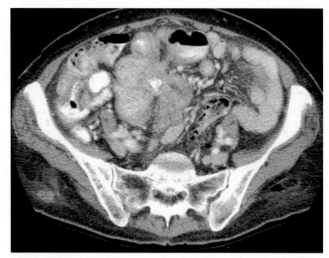

FIGURE 2.8B

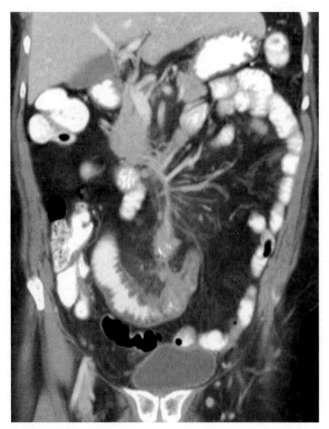

FIGURE 2.8C

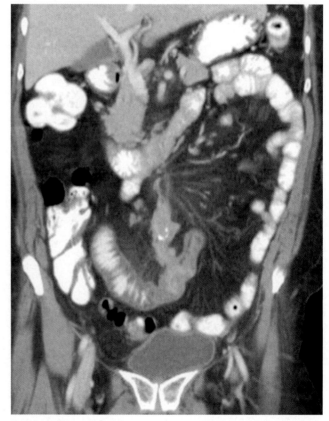

FIGURE 2.8D

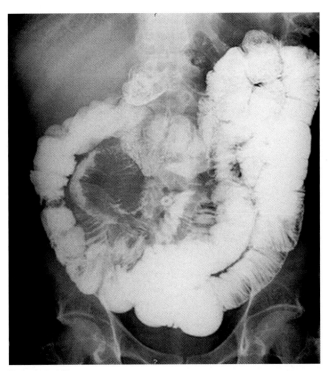

FIGURE 2.8E

FINDINGS CT image through the liver (A) obtained in the arterial phase of enhancement demonstrates at least five hyperenhancing liver lesions. CT image obtained through the lower abdomen (B) demonstrates a calcified right lower quadrant mesenteric mass with tethering of adjacent small bowel loops that are also thick walled. Coronal reformations from a second patient demonstrate a calcified mesenteric mass extending into distal ileum (C, D). The distal ileum is also thick walled (C, D). Small bowel follow-through (E) demonstrates tethering of small bowel loops in the right lower abdomen.

DIFFERENTIAL DIAGNOSIS Metastatic carcinoid tumor.

DIAGNOSIS Metastatic carcinoid tumor.

DISCUSSION Carcinoid tumors can be classified as foregut (20% to 25%, including lung, thymus, stomach, and proximal duodenum), midgut (40% to 50%, including distal duodenum, small bowel, appendix, and proximal colon), and hindgut (15%, including distal colon and rectum). Carcinoid tumors are generally relatively slow growing. Even with metastatic disease, 5-year survival is 70% to 80%.

At CT, mesenteric masses related to carcinoid tumors are calcified in approximately 70% of cases. These mesenteric masses are metastases, typically from an ileal tumor which is often small, occult at imaging, and may be multifocal. Serotonin and other substances released by these tumors can trigger a desmoplastic reaction in the mesentery. This desmoplastic reaction can compress mesenteric veins resulting in bowel wall thickening as in this case.

Liver metastases are usually hypervascular and therefore best appreciated in the arterial phase of imaging (approximately 20 seconds after contrast administration). Bone metastases from carcinoid tumors are typically sclerotic.

Questions for Further Thought

1. Although most carcinoid tumors are sporadic, they can be associated with syndromes. Name three such syndromes.
2. Name symptoms associated with carcinoid syndrome.

Reporting Responsibilities

1. Describe the sites of metastatic disease (most frequently small bowel mesentery and liver for GI carcinoid tumors).
2. Attempt to identify the site of the primary tumor. However, primary GI carcinoid tumors are frequently so small that they are occult at imaging.

What the Treating Physician Needs to Know

1. When carcinoid tumor is suspected, correlation with urine levels of 5-hydroxyindoleacetic acid (a breakdown product of serotonin) can help confirm the diagnosis.
2. ^{111}In-octreotide scintigraphy is frequently used for staging of carcinoid tumors.

Answers

1. Syndromes associated with carcinoid tumors include multiple endocrine neoplasia (MEN) type 1, MEN type 2, and neurofibromatosis type 1.
2. Symptoms associated with carcinoid syndrome include diarrhea, abdominal cramping, and facial and upper body flushing. Carcinoid syndrome implies the presence of liver metastases.

REFERENCES

1. Scarsbrook AF, Ganeshan A, Statham J, et al. Anatomic and functional imaging of metastatic carcinoid tumors. Radiographics 2007;27:455-477.
2. Kulke MH, Mayer RJ. Carcinoid tumors. N Engl J Med 1999;340:858-868.

CLINICAL HISTORY *21-year-old man with abdominal pain.*

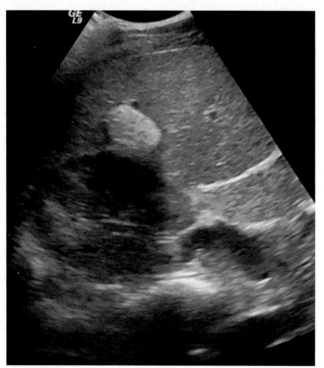

FIGURE 2.9A

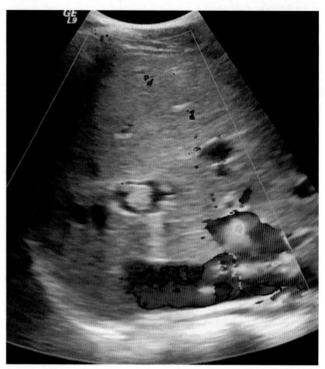

FIGURE 2.9B

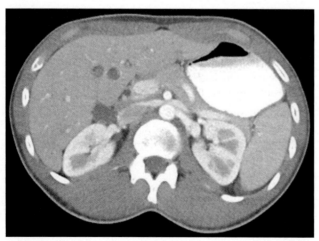

FIGURE 2.9C

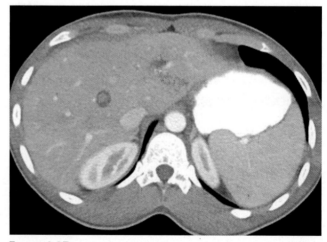

FIGURE 2.9D

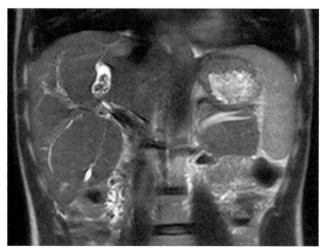

FIGURE 2.9E

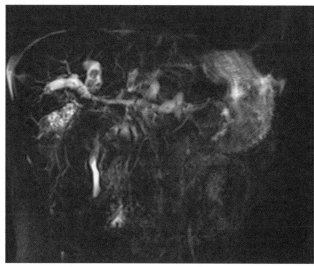

FIGURE 2.9F

FINDINGS Grayscale US (A) demonstrates a 2.7-cm intrahepatic echogenic, shadowing structure in keeping with a stone. Color Doppler US (B) in a different area of the liver demonstrates an additional echogenic shadowing structure surrounded by anechoic material. Note also intrahepatic biliary ductal dilatation (B). Contrast-enhanced CT (C, D) demonstrates intrahepatic high attenuation structures surrounded by low attenuation fluid. T2-weighted coronal MR image (E) demonstrates that the echogenic, high attenuation structures seen in (A) to (D) are stones within a dilated intrahepatic biliary system. Slab MRCP image (F) demonstrates moderate intrahepatic biliary ductal dilatation. In summary, this patient has numerous stones within a dilated intrahepatic biliary system.

DIFFERENTIAL DIAGNOSIS Recurrent pyogenic cholangitis (RPC).

DIAGNOSIS RPC.

DISCUSSION Patients with RPC have intrahepatic biliary strictures, which lead to irregular intrahepatic biliary ductal dilatation, bile stasis, and eventual pigment stone formation. Strictures of the extrahepatic biliary system are uncommon. Pigment stones are hypointense (black) at T2-weighted imaging and may have intrinsic T1 bright signal. The left hepatic lobe is affected more often than the right, but bilobar involvement is also common.

If bile ducts are acutely infected or inflamed, wall hyperemia may be seen at arterial phase MR imaging. Intrahepatic abscesses may occur in up to 20% of patients. Over time, portal vein thrombosis and eventual parenchymal atrophy may develop.

Patients often experience repeated episodes of cholangitis due to superimposed infection and may present with fever, right upper quadrant pain, and jaundice. The infectious organism in the acute setting is usually bacteria. *Clonorchis sinensis* and *Ascaris lumbricoides* infestation have also been found in patients with RPC, but a direct link between the two conditions has not been established definitively.

RPC has also been described by a number of other names such as oriental cholangiohepatitis and hepatolithiasis. Although previously thought to be more common in the Far East, the prevalence of RPC is thought to be increasing in western countries.

Questions for Further Thought

1. True or false: Patients with RPC are at increased risk for cholangiocarcinoma?
2. What is the management of RPC?

Reporting Responsibilities

1. Evaluate for acute complications such as intrahepatic abscess formation.
2. Describe the distribution of ductal dilatation and stricturing as well as the distribution of stones as this information will help guide long-term management (see answer 2 below).

What the Treating Physician Needs to Know

1. Patients with RPC are at increased risk for cholangiocarcinoma. Routine follow-up imaging should be considered for cholangiocarcinoma screening.

Answers

1. True. Patients with RPC are at increased risk for cholangiocarcinoma.
2. In the acute setting, management includes antibiotics, endoscopic or radiologic biliary drainage, and supportive care. Long-term management goals include removing ductal stones (e.g., via endoscopic retrograde cholangiopancreatography (ERCP) or surgically) and dilating strictured areas when possible. Depending on disease burden, surgical biliary exploration with stone clearance, choledochojejunostomy, or hepatic lobar resection may be required.

REFERENCES

1. Park M-S, Yu J-S, Kim KW, et al. Recurrent pyogenic cholangitis: comparison between MR cholangiography and direct cholangiography. Radiology 2002;220:677-682.
2. Catalano OA, Sahani DV, Forcione DG. Biliary infections: spectrum of imaging findings and management. Radiology 2009;29:2059-2080.

CLINICAL HISTORY *65-year-old man with worsening abdominal pain 2 days following laparoscopic cholecystectomy.*

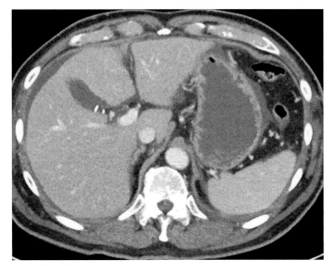

FIGURE 2.10A

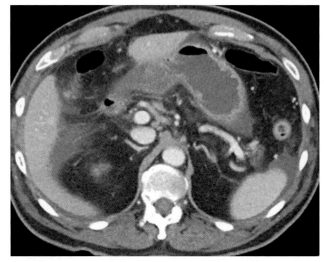

FIGURE 2.10B

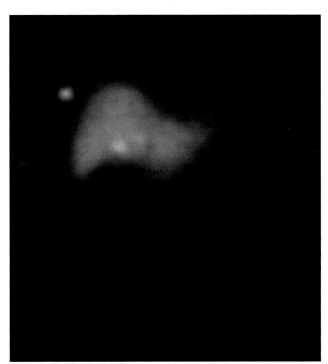

FIGURE 2.10C

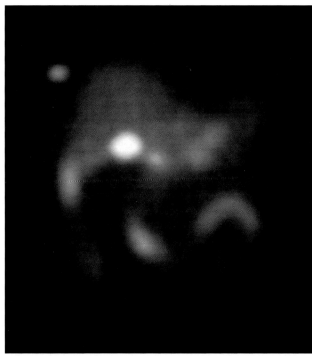

FIGURE 2.10D

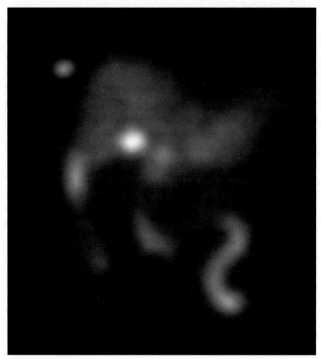

FIGURE 2.10E

FINDINGS Contrast-enhanced CT demonstrates surgical clips in the gallbladder fossa along with fluid (A). Fluid is also present around the liver, stomach, and spleen (A, B). Hepatobiliary iminodiacetic acid (HIDA) scan demonstrates normal hepatic uptake of the radiopharmaceutical approximately 2 minutes post injection (C). In the 30-minute image (D), radiopharmaceutical is visible accumulating in the gallbladder fossa and also tracking around the liver including extending down the right paracolic gutter. In the 60-minute image (E), increased accumulation is seen along the right paracolic gutter.

DIFFERENTIAL DIAGNOSIS (BASED ON CT) Ascites, bile duct leak.

DIAGNOSIS Bile duct leak.

DISCUSSION Bile duct leaks occur in <1% of patients following laparoscopic cholecystectomy. The perihepatic fluid visible in the above CT images is nonspecific but is suspicious for a bile duct leak in an otherwise healthy patient following cholecystectomy. Ascites, for example due to liver disease, could have a similar appearance in the appropriate clinical setting. A small amount of fluid is not unexpected in the gallbladder fossa following cholecystectomy, but fluid should not be visible surrounding the liver and spleen in an otherwise healthy patient.

The above HIDA scan images are diagnostic of a bile duct leak as radiopharmaceutical is seen accumulating in the gallbladder fossa and tracking along the right paracolic gutter. Normally the radiopharmaceutical is excreted by the liver into the common bile duct and duodenum and then advances through the rest of the small and large intestines.

Bile duct leaks may be due to leakage from the cystic duct stump, injury to the hepatic duct, or to disruption of accessory hepatic ducts that drain from the liver parenchyma directly into the gallbladder. Such accessory ducts occur in 5% to 6% of individuals at autopsy and if identified during surgery are usually clipped.

Other complications of cholecystectomy include bile duct occlusion and gallstone spillage. Bile duct occlusion is usually due to accidental clipping of the main hepatic duct, right duct, or left duct during surgery. At imaging, occluded bile ducts typically appear "dry" manifesting as ductal dilatation without significant associated perihepatic fluid.

Question for Further Thought

1. What is the usual management of a bile leak?

Reporting Requirements

1. Based on the CT, report the presence of perihepatic fluid that is suspicious for a bile leak.
2. Suggest a HIDA scan or MR study with a hepatobiliary contrast agent and delayed imaging for further evaluation. HIDA scan can confirm the presence of a leak. The superior soft tissue resolution of MR can often identify the site of the leak.

What the Treating Physician Needs to Know

1. This patient has generalized free fluid in the upper abdomen that is suspicious for a bile leak following cholecystectomy.

Answer

1. Bile leaks are often managed with CT- or US-guided placement of a drainage catheter into the fluid. A stent may be placed across the common bile duct via ERCP. Bile leaks usually heal with this type of minimally invasive approach.

REFERENCES

1. Duca S, Bala O, Al-Hajjar N, Iancu C, Puia IC, Munteanu D, Graur F. Laparoscopic cholecystectomy: incidence and complications. A retrospective analysis of 9542 consecutive laparoscopic operations. HPB 2003;5:152-158.
2. Ahmad F, Saunders RN, Lloyd GM, Lloyd DM, Robertson GSM. An algorithm for the management of bile leak following laparoscopic cholecystectomy. Ann R Coll Surg Engl 2007; 89:5-56.

CLINICAL HISTORY *53-year-old woman, history withheld.*

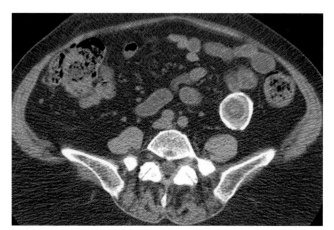

FIGURE 2.11A

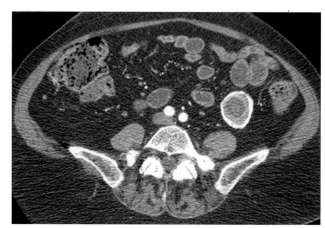

FIGURE 2.11B

FINDINGS Noncontrast CT (A) demonstrates a 3 cm calcified structure in the left abdomen without adjacent inflammatory change. No enhancement is visible in the postcontrast image (B).

DIFFERENTIAL DIAGNOSIS Calcified loose body due to prior episode of epiploic appendagitis, calcified lymph node, dropped gallstone.

DIAGNOSIS Dropped gallstone.

DISCUSSION The lamellated pattern of calcification in the above case is characteristic of a gallstone. Gallstone spillage occurs fairly commonly in patients undergoing laparoscopic cholecystectomy with spill rates of 6% to 30% in some series. Dropped gallstones are thought to more commonly occur during laparoscopic as compared with open cholecystectomies. Dropped stones may be located within the abdominal cavity or within subcutaneous tissues at a port site. Case reports of dropped gallstones appearing in urine and sputum have been described.

Fortunately, complications from dropped gallstones are rare occurring in <1% of patients. The most common complication is abscess formation with patients presenting an average of 4 months after cholecystectomy. Patients presenting with abscess due to a dropped gallstone between 1 month and 20 years following cholecystectomy have been described.

As compared with the lamellated appearance of the above stone, calcified lymph nodes usually demonstrate dense, chunky calcifications. Calcified lymph nodes often reflect prior granulomatous disease (e.g., histoplasmosis or tuberculosis).

Calcified loose bodies due to a prior episode of epiploic appendagitis usually appear as ovoid or round dense calcifications and are most commonly located in the dependent pelvis. When epiploic appendages torse and undergo infarction, they may detach from the colon and eventually calcify becoming calcified loose bodies.

Question for Further Thought

1. What is the usual treatment of a dropped gallstone?

Reporting Requirements

1. Describe the presence of a dropped gallstone.
2. Evaluate for evidence of infection such as inflammatory changes or a fluid collection associated with a dropped gallstone.

What the Treating Physician Needs to Know

1. The size and location of the dropped stone.
2. If there is evidence of associated infection or abscess formation.

Answer

1. During the initial cholecystectomy, attempts are made to remove all dropped gallstones. If a dropped stone is detected at imaging following the initial surgery, management depends on patient symptomatology and whether or not inflammatory changes are visible around the stone at imaging. Noninfected stones are usually left alone. Infected stones may be removed. Removal techniques include removal with a nephroscope via a small incision. Stone size impacts potential removal options.

REFERENCES

1. Morrin MM, Kruskal JB, Hochman MG, Saldinger PF, Kane RA. Radiologic features of complications arising from dropped gallstones in laparoscopic cholecystectomy patients. Am J Roentgenol 2000;174:1441-1445.
2. Sathesh-Kumar T, Saklani AP, Vinayagam R, Blackett RL. Review: spilled gallstones during laparoscopic cholecystectomy: a review of the literature. Postgrad Med J 2004;80:77-79.

CLINICAL HISTORY *34-year-old man with abdominal pain (A, B) and 32-year-old woman with abdominal pain (C, D).*

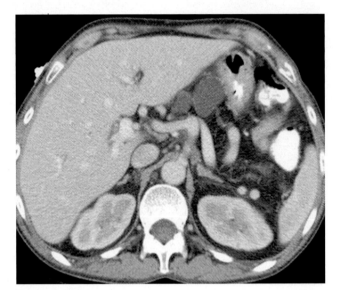

FIGURE 2.12A

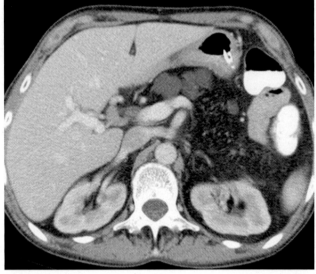

FIGURE 2.12B

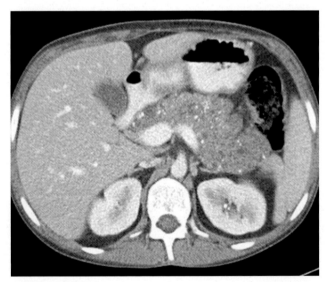

FIGURE 2.12C

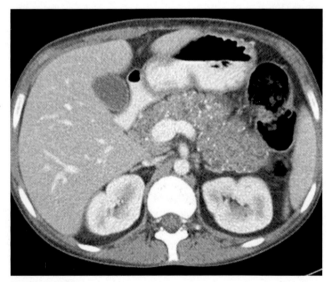

FIGURE 2.12D

FINDINGS CT images obtained with intravenous and oral contrast material demonstrate fatty replacement of the pancreas and multiple fluid attenuation masses in the pancreatic bed measuring up to 3 cm (A, B). In the second patient, the pancreas is diffusely enlarged by innumerable small cystic structures (C, D). Scattered calcifications are also present (C, D). Both patients have cystic fibrosis.

DIFFERENTIAL DIAGNOSIS Abscesses, necrotic lymph nodes, pancreatic cystosis, von Hippel Lindau (VHL) disease.

DIAGNOSIS Pancreatic cystosis associated with cystic fibrosis.

DISCUSSION The cysts of cystic fibrosis associated pancreatic cystosis are true epithelial lined cysts that are thought to form as a result of inspissated secretions leading to ductal ectasia. These cysts are not thought to have any malignant potential.

The key to the diagnosis in this case is realizing that the pancreas is entirely fatty replaced as is seen with cystic fibrosis. The cystic structures in this case are entirely cystic and have no surrounding inflammatory changes. Abscesses would be expected to demonstrate adjacent inflammatory changes. Necrotic lymph nodes would have a solid component. Renal cysts along with pancreatic cysts would be expected in a patient with VHL disease.

Questions for Further Thought

1. Do you think the pancreatic cysts are the cause of this patient's abdominal pain?
2. What is the treatment for pancreatic cystosis?

Reporting Responsibilities

1. Confidently make the diagnosis of pancreatic cystosis when multiple pancreatic cysts are seen in a patient with cystic fibrosis.

What the Treating Physician Needs to Know

1. The diagnosis of pancreatic cystosis can be made with confidence in a patient with cystic fibrosis and usually does not require tissue confirmation.

Answers

1. Pancreatic cystosis is a rare entity with a few cases reported in the literature. No standard treatment protocol for this condition exists. Case reports have described patients with cystic fibrosis associated pancreatic cystosis and debilitating abdominal pain that resolved with pancreatectomy. Alternatively, other case reports have described patients with cystic fibrosis associated pancreatic cystosis with no significant abdominal pain.

2. Treatment depends on the patient's symptoms and whether the symptoms are thought to be due to pancreatic pathology. Reported treatments range from doing nothing to pancreatectomy.

REFERENCES

1. Hernanz-Schulman M, Teele RL, Perez-Atayde A, et al. Pancreatic cystosis in cystic fibrosis. Radiology 1986;158: 629-631.
2. van Rijn RR, Schilte PP, Wiarda BM, et al. Case 113: pancreatic cystosis. Radiology 2007;243:598-602.

CLINICAL HISTORY *23-year-old woman with abdominal pain.*

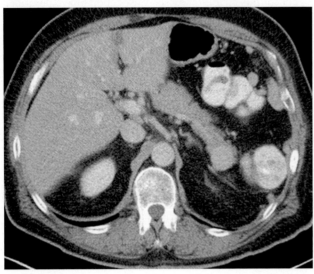

FIGURE 2.13A

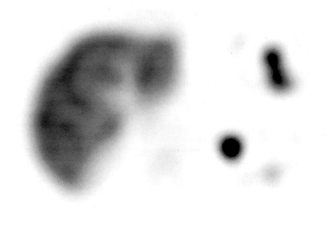

FIGURE 2.13B

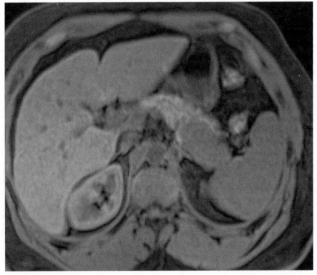

FIGURE 2.13C

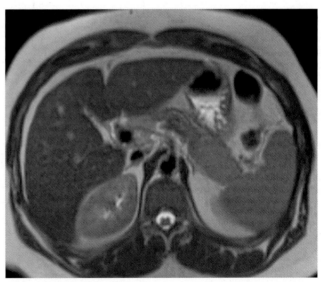

FIGURE 2.13D

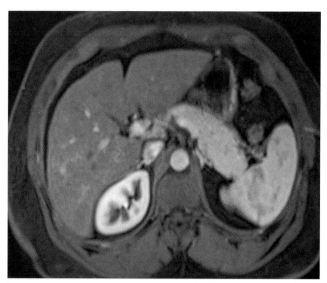

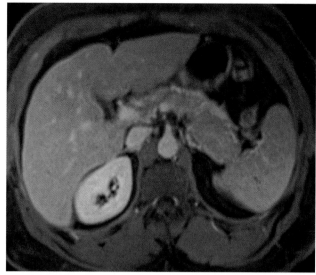

FIGURE 2.13E

FIGURE 2.13F

FINDINGS (A) CT with contrast demonstrates a 2-cm round hyperenhancing mass in the pancreatic tail. (B) Discussed in discussion below. Images (C) to (F) are from a different patient with the same diagnosis and demonstrate a 3.5-cm ovoid mass in the pancreatic tail. This mass demonstrates T1 dark signal (C) and T2 dark signal (D) that is similar to the signal intensity of the spleen. The mass also enhances similar to spleen during the arterial (E) and portal venous (F) phases of enhancement.

DIFFERENTIAL DIAGNOSIS Hypervascular metastasis, intrapancreatic splenule, islet cell tumor.

DIAGNOSIS Intrapancreatic splenule.

DISCUSSION Intrapancreatic splenule should be considered in the differential diagnosis of a hyperenhancing mass in the pancreatic tail. Intrapancreatic splenules account for approximately 20% of accessory spleens.

At CT, the enhancement of an intrapancreatic splenule matches that of the spleen. At MR, the signal intensity of an intrapancreatic splenule follows the spleen on all pulse sequences.

Intrapancreatic splenules can appear very similar to islet cell tumors and hypervascular metastases. The most helpful clues to the diagnosis of an intrapancreatic splenule are (1) characteristic location in the pancreatic tail and (2) attenuation or signal intensity which follows the spleen. Often the diagnosis of intrapancreatic splenule can be made with CT or MR, but up to 30% of intrapancreatic splenules may hypoenhance relative to the spleen and therefore be difficult to diagnose.

In cases in which the diagnosis of an intrapancreatic splenule cannot be made with confidence at CT or MR, ^{99m}Tc-sulfur colloid scan or a damaged red blood cell scan are noninvasive ways to confirm the diagnosis. The above patient underwent a ^{99m}Tc-sulfur colloid scan (B). Note the accumulation of the radiopharmaceutical in the pancreatic tail at a location corresponding to the hyperenhancing pancreatic tail mass seen at CT. Note also the accumulation of radiopharmaceutical in the left anterior abdomen where the patient also has other splenules that were visible at CT. The nuclear medicine study was diagnostic of an intrapancreatic splenule, and tissue sampling was not necessary.

Question for Further Thought

1. What are other potential locations of accessory spleens?

Reporting Requirements

1. Describe the size and location of the mass.
2. When possible, make the diagnosis of intrapancreatic splenule at CT or MR.
3. If an intrapancreatic splenule is suspected, but the diagnosis cannot be made with absolute confidence at CT or MR, ^{99m}Tc-sulfur colloid scan or a damaged red blood cell scan are noninvasive ways to confirm the diagnosis.

What the Treating Physician Needs to Know

1. This patient has a pancreatic tail mass which is suggestive of an intrapancreatic splenule.
2. The diagnosis of an intrapancreatic splenule is confirmed in the ^{99m}Tc-sulfur colloid scan.

Answer

1. Accessory spleens may be located in a variety of locations, including adjacent to the spleen, in the gastrosplenic ligament, in the splenorenal ligament, in the mesentery, in the pelvis, or even in the chest following trauma.

REFERENCES

1. Sica GT, Reed MF. Case 27: intrapancreatic accessory spleen. Radiology 2000;217:134-137.
2. Mortele KJ, Mortele B, Silverman SG. CT features of accessory spleen. Am J Roentgenol 2004;183:1653-1657.

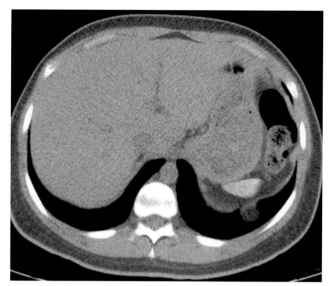

FIGURE 2.14A

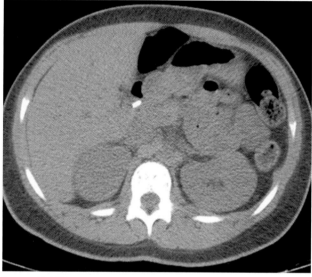

FIGURE 2.14B

FINDINGS Noncontrast CT images demonstrate an approximately 4-cm calcified structure in the left upper quadrant (A). Surgical clips are visible in the gallbladder fossa (B).

DIFFERENTIAL DIAGNOSIS Autoinfarcted spleen, calcified granulomas.

DIAGNOSIS Autoinfarcted spleen in the setting of sickle cell disease.

DISCUSSION Sickle cell anemia is characterized by abnormal red blood cell morphology due to abnormal hemoglobin. These abnormally shaped red blood cells are rapidly removed from circulation, resulting in anemia. Sickle cell anemia occurs in approximately 1 in 375 African-American individuals in the United States.

The abnormally shaped red blood cells in individuals with sickle cell anemia can, through sluggish flow, result in tissue infarction in a variety of locations, including the bone marrow, brain, chest, abdomen, and pelvis. The spleen is especially prone to infarction due to its sluggish blood flow. By age 5, approximately 94% of individuals with sickle cell anemia have auto-infarcted spleens and are functionally asplenic. Patients who are functionally asplenic are prone to infection and may require prophylactic antibiotics.

At CT, splenic autoinfarction manifests as a small, calcified spleen. By comparison, calcified splenic granulomas appear as discrete, rounded splenic calcifications usually

measuring less than 1 cm in size. The cholecystectomy clips in the above case are an additional diagnostic clue as patients with sickle cell disease often develop pigment gallstones and eventually undergo cholecystectomy. At MR, autoinfarcted spleens demonstrate low signal on all pulse sequences.

Questions for Further Thought

1. What other manifestations of sickle cell disease may be visible at abdominopelvic CT?
2. Name another splenic manifestation of sickle cell disease.

Reporting Requirements

1. Describe the presence of a small calcified spleen indicating an autoinfarcted spleen.
2. Evaluate for other findings of sickle cell disease (see below).

What the Treating Physician Needs to Know

1. A small calcified spleen usually reflects an autoinfarcted spleen in a patient with sickle cell anemia.

Answers

1. Patients with sickle cell disease may demonstrate dense bones, H-shaped or Lincoln log vertebral bodies (due to bone infarcts), avascular necrosis of the femoral heads, gallstones, renal papillary necrosis, and a hyperattenuating liver due to hemosiderosis from multiple blood transfusions. Rarely, extramedullary hematopoiesis may

involve the solid abdominal organs, including the liver, spleen, and adrenal glands. Extramedullary hematopoiesis manifests as hypoenhancing masses and can be confirmed with ^{99m}Tc-sulfur colloid imaging.

2. Patients with sickle cell disease may develop splenic sequestration, a potentially life-threatening condition characterized by pooling of red blood cells in the spleen with resultant tachycardia and hypotension in severe cases. At imaging, splenic sequestration manifests as splenic enlargement and heterogeneity.

REFERENCE

1. Lonergan GJ, Cline DB, Abbondanzo SL. Sickle cell anemia. Radiographics 2001;21:971-994.

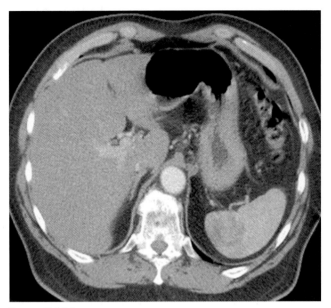

FIGURE 2.15A

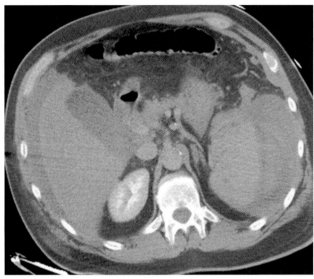

FIGURE 2.15B

FINDINGS Initial contrast-enhanced CT image (A) demonstrates subtle heterogeneity of the posterior spleen indicating splenic contusion. Two days later, the patient developed acute onset abdominal pain, tachycardia, and hypotension with contrast-enhanced CT (B) demonstrating large volume blood products around the liver and the spleen.

DIAGNOSIS Delayed splenic rupture.

DISCUSSION Management options for severe splenic injuries include splenectomy and embolization. Evidence of active bleeding is an indication for splenectomy or embolization. However, for patients with more minor splenic injuries, conservative non-invasive management is preferred as preservation of splenic tissue decreases the risk of later infectious complications.

Delayed splenic rupture is a potential complication of conservative management of splenic injuries. Delayed splenic bleeding or rupture occurs in approximately 10% of patients with splenic injuries. 75% of delayed splenic ruptures occur within two days of the initial injury, and more than 90% of delayed ruptures occur within the first week. A proposed mechanism for delayed splenic rupture is lysis of clot, increased intraparenchymal pressure, and resultant new bleeding.

Questions for Further Thought

1. What is the most commonly injured solid abdominal organ?

Reporting Requirement for Initial Scan (A)

1. Describe the presence of a splenic contusion.

What the Treating Physician Needs to Know

1. Patients with splenic injuries that are managed conservatively are at risk for delayed splenic rupture. Such patients should be warned of this possibility at discharge and instructed to return to the hospital if they develop symptoms of bleeding such as abdominal pain.

Answer

1. The spleen is the most commonly injured solid abdominal organ.

REFERENCES

1. McIntyre LK, Schiff MS, Jurkovich GJ. Failure of nonoperative management of splenic injuries. Arch Surg 2005;140:563-569.
2. Crawford RS, Tabbara M, Sheridan R, Spaniolas KG, Velmahos GC. Early discharge after nonoperative management for splenic injuries: increased patient risk caused by late failure? Surgery 2007;142:337-342.

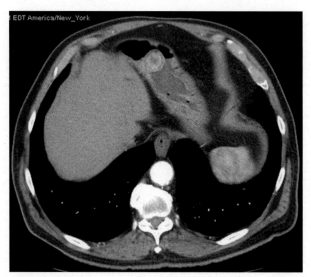

FIGURE 2.16A

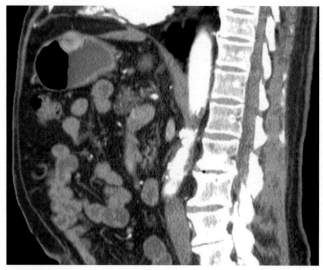

FIGURE 2.16B

FINDINGS Axial (A) and sagittal (B) contrast-enhanced CT images demonstrate a 2.5-cm well-circumscribed round enhancing mass arising from the wall of the distal gastric body.

DIFFERENTIAL DIAGNOSIS Gastric adenocarcinoma, Gastrointestinal stromal tumor (GIST).

DIAGNOSIS GIST.

DISCUSSION The well-circumscribed nature of this mass is characteristic of a submucosal mass. GIST is the most common submucosal gastric mass, and the stomach is the most common location for a GIST. Other less common submucosal masses that can occur in the stomach are lipoma, leiomyoma, neuroma, fibroma, and neurofibroma. Lipomas demonstrate uniform low attenuation at CT (negative Hounsfield units) since they are composed entirely of fat. The other listed submucosal masses will all appear as soft-tissue masses and usually require tissue sampling for diagnosis.

By comparison, when visible at CT gastric adenocarcinoma usually appears as a more ill-defined mass that infiltrates along the gastric wall rather than a well-circumscribed round mass as in the above case. Keep in mind that routine CT is an insensitive test for the detection of small gastric cancers.

Questions for Further Thought

1. What is the usual management of a gastric GIST?
2. Are GISTs thought to have malignant potential?

Reporting Requirements

1. Describe the size and location of the mass.
2. Report that imaging features favor a submucosal mass, statistically most likely a GIST.

What the Treating Physician Needs to Know

1. This patient has a 2.5-cm gastric mass that is statistically most likely a GIST.

Answers

1. Gastric GISTs are usually resected.
2. GISTs are thought to have malignant potential. The liver is the most common site of metastatic disease.

REFERENCE

1. American Gastroenterological Association Institute technical review on the management of gastric subepithelial masses. Gastroenterology 2006;130:2217-2228.

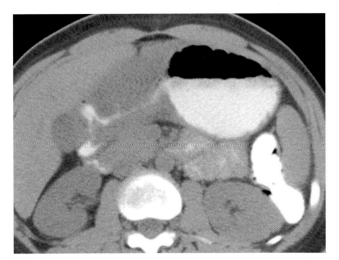

FIGURE 2.17A

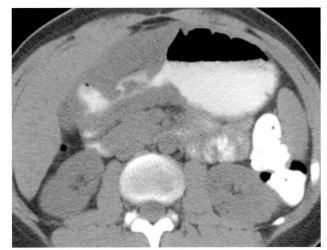

FIGURE 2.17B

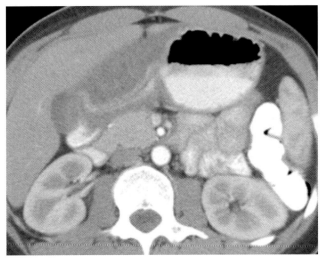

FIGURE 2.17C

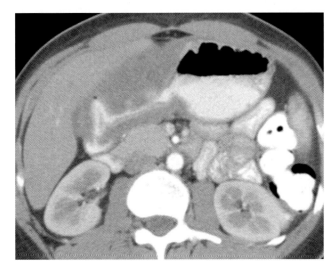

FIGURE 2.17D

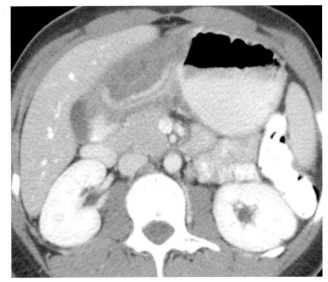

FIGURE 2.17E

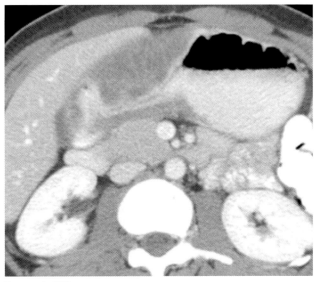

FIGURE 2.17F

FINDINGS Noncontrast (A, B), arterial phase (C, D), and portal venous phase (E, F) CT images demonstrate marked hypoenhancing circumferential wall thickening of the gastric antrum.

DIFFERENTIAL DIAGNOSIS Adenocarcinoma, lymphoma.

DIAGNOSIS Adenocarcinoma.

DISCUSSION Adenocarcinomas account for more than 95% of malignant gastric tumors. At CT, gastric adenocarcinomas appear as segmental or diffuse areas of gastric wall thickening. Lymphoma can also appear as segmental or diffuse wall gastric thickening but is much less common than gastric adenocarcinoma. Lymphoma is more commonly multifocal as compared with adenocarcinoma.

Adequate distention of the stomach is necessary to accurately diagnose pathologic wall thickening. For example, when the stomach is collapsed it often appears thick walled. "Shouldering" is a helpful clue to distinguish pathologic from physiologic wall thickening and is demonstrated in the above case. "Shouldering" is defined as an abrupt transition from normal thickness bowel wall to the area of wall thickening. Detection of subtle tumors also is improved with the use of water as a negative oral contrast agent as compared with positive contrast agents such as iodine- or barium-based agents.

Question for Further Thought

1. What would be a reasonable protocol for administration of water (a negative contrast agent) to achieve adequate distention of the stomach to evaluate for gastric cancer?

Reporting Requirement

1. Describe the presence and location of wall thickening that is suspicious for malignancy.

What the Treating Physician Needs to Know

1. Tissue sampling will likely be needed to establish the diagnosis in this patient.

Answer

1. According to Horton et al.,[1] 750 mL of water should be administered approximately 15 minutes prior to the scan with 250 mL of water ingested immediately prior to imaging.

REFERENCE

1. Horton KM, Fishman EK. Current role of CT in imaging of the stomach. Radiographics 2003;23:75-87.

CLINICAL HISTORY *67-year-old man with a history of aortobifemoral bypass graft, abdominal pain, fever, and malaise.*

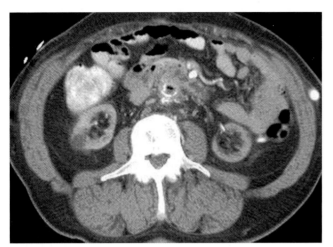

FIGURE 2.18A

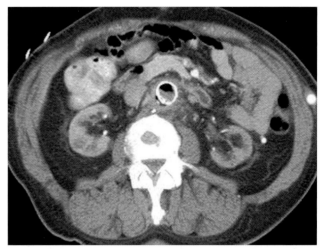

FIGURE 2.18B

FINDINGS Contrast-enhanced CT images demonstrate wall thickening of the third portion of the duodenum (A) and loss of fat plane around the aorta with periaortic fat stranding (B). Note air in the lumen of the patient's aortic graft.

DIFFERENTIAL DIAGNOSIS Aortoenteric fistula, aortic/peri-aortic infection without fistulization.

DIAGNOSIS Aortoenteric fistula.

DISCUSSION CT findings specific for an aortoenteric fistula include extravasation of intravenous contrast material from the aorta into bowel, ectopic air located around or within the aorta more than 4 weeks after aortic surgery, and leakage of oral contrast material around the aorta. If GI bleeding is the chief complaint, inflammatory changes around the aorta could also indicate an aortoenteric fistula. Angiography may demonstrate leakage of contrast material from the aorta into the bowel, though the absence of this finding does not exclude a fistula.

A primary aortoenteric fistula is defined as a direct communication between the aorta and the bowel in a patient with no prior aortic surgery and is most commonly seen in patients with abdominal aortic aneurysms or aortic infections.

A secondary aortoenteric fistula is defined as a communication between the aorta and the bowel in a patient with prior aortic surgery. Secondary fistulas are more common than primary fistulas, and the majority of these fistulas involve the third or fourth portions of the duodenum.

Based on CT findings of aortoenteric fistula, the patient was taken to the operating room where a secondary aortoenteric

fistula between the grafted portion of the aorta and the third portion of the duodenum was confirmed and repaired.

Questions for Further Thought

1. What are treatment options for aortoenteric fistulas?
2. What symptoms are associated with aortoenteric fistulas?

Reporting Responsibilities

1. When specific signs of an aortoenteric fistula as noted above are present, the diagnosis can be made with CT.
2. The ordering clinician should be contacted immediately with this critical finding.

What the Treating Physician Needs to Know

1. An aortoenteric fistula is a surgical emergency and a vascular surgeon should be consulted immediately.

Answers

1. Historically, resection with bypass grafting was the preferred treatment for aortoenteric fistulas. More recently, covered aortic stent grafts have been used to repair aortoenteric fistulas.
2. Symptoms may include abdominal pain, low-grade fevers, and GI bleeding, which may be small volume and intermittent ("herald bleeds") or catastrophic.

REFERENCES

1. Vu QDM, Menias CO, Bhalla S, Peterson C, et al. Aortoenteric fistulas: CT features and potential mimics. Radiographics 2009;29:197-209.
2. Verhey P, Best A, Lakin P, Nachiondo J, Peterson B. Successful endovascular treatment of aortoenteric fistula secondary to eroding duodenal stent. J Vasc Interv Radiol 2006;17:1345-1348.

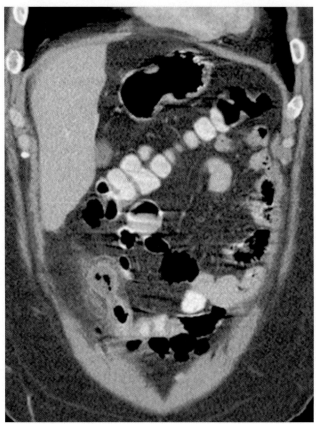

FIGURE 2.19

FINDINGS Coronal reformation CT image obtained after administration of intravenous and oral contrast material demonstrates a blind-ending tubular structure in the right lower quadrant with surrounding inflammatory changes.

DIFFERENTIAL DIAGNOSIS Acute appendicitis, Meckel diverticulitis.

DIAGNOSIS Meckel diverticulitis.

DISCUSSION A Meckel diverticulum results from failure of atrophy of the omphalomesenteric duct. These diverticula are found in 2% to 3% of the population but become symptomatic only in a minority of people.

Patients with an inflamed Meckel diverticulum may present with symptoms that mimic acute appendicitis. The key to making the correct imaging diagnosis is determining from where the blind-ending tubular structure arises. The appendix arises from the base of the cecum. By comparison, a Meckel diverticulum arises from the ileum, usually within 2 feet of the ileocecal valve. Meckel diverticula can be difficult to identify at CT, especially in patients with scant intra-abdominal fat.

Meckel diverticula sometimes contain heterotopic gastric and pancreatic mucosa. A ^{99m}Tc pertechnetate scan can be used to detect Meckel diverticula that contain ectopic gastric mucosa.

A hernia containing a Meckel diverticulum is called a Littre hernia.

Questions for Further Thought

1. What is the most common complication of a Meckel diverticulum?
2. What is the treatment of a symptomatic Meckel diverticulum?

Reporting Responsibilities

1. Distinguish a Meckel diverticulum from the appendix.
2. Describe any complications such as a diverticulitis and bowel obstruction.

What the Treating Physician Needs to Know

1. Unlike this case, in most individuals Meckel diverticula are often difficult to identify at CT. If there is strong clinical suspicion, a ^{99m}Tc pertechnetate scan should be considered.

Answers

1. Bleeding due to ulceration of heterotopic gastric mucosa is the most common complication of a Meckel diverticulum.
2. Surgical resection is the treatment of choice for a symptomatic Meckel diverticulum.

REFERENCE

1. Levy AD, Hobbs CM. From the archives of the AFIP Meckel diverticulum: radiologic features with pathologic correlation. Radiographics 2004;24:565-587.

CLINICAL HISTORY *62-year-old man with nausea, vomiting, and diarrhea.*

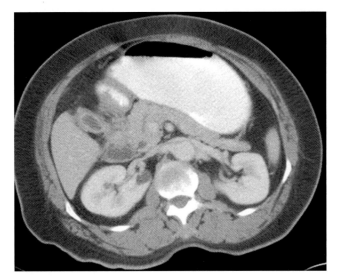

FIGURE 2.20A

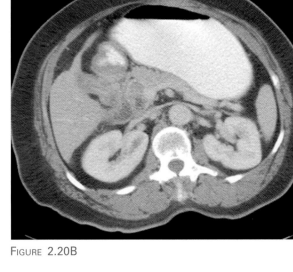

FIGURE 2.20B

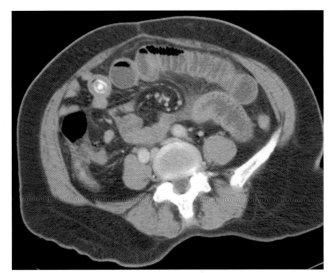

FIGURE 2.20C

FINDINGS Contrast-enhanced CT images obtained after administration of intravenous and oral contrast material demonstrate a distended stomach (A, B) with dilated small bowel loops (C). An approximately 2.5-cm lamellated calcified structure is visible within a small bowel loop in the right lower quadrant (C). Dilated small bowel loops lead up to this calcified structure, and decompressed small bowel loops lead away from it. The patient's gallbladder is decompressed but demonstrates mucosal hyperemia (A, B).

DIAGNOSIS Gallstone ileus.

DISCUSSION The distended stomach and dilated loops of small bowel visible in this patient indicate a small bowel obstruction. When evaluating a patient with a small bowel obstruction, dilated small bowel loops should be traced distally until the transition point to decompressed small bowel loops is identified.

The transition point should be interrogated for potential etiologies such as a hernia or mass. In the above case, a calcified gallstone was identified at the transition point which is diagnostic of a gallstone ileus. (If no cause of obstruction is identified at the transition point, adhesions should be assumed. Adhesions, the most common cause of small bowel obstruction, usually are not discretely visible at CT.)

The term "gallstone ileus" is a misnomer as this condition is usually a mechanical small bowel obstruction due to gallstone impaction. Gallstone ileus most common occurs in elderly persons. The impacted gallstone usually reaches the small intestine via a fistulous communication between gallbladder and small intestine.

When evaluating a patient with suspected gallstone ileus, the gallbladder should be evaluated to see if a residual fistulous tract is visible. Additionally, the intestinal tract should be interrogated for other large gallstones that could be other potential sources of obstruction. Air is often visible in the biliary system in patients with gallstone ileus and enters the biliary system via fistulous communication with bowel.

Questions for Further Thought

1. What is Rigler triad?
2. What is the usual treatment for gallstone ileus?

Reporting Requirements

1. Describe the presence of a gallstone in the distal small intestine resulting in a small bowel obstruction.
2. Report any additional large gallstones visible in the GI tract.
3. Evaluate for a visible fistula between the gallbladder and the bowel.

What the Treating Physician Needs to Know

1. This patient has a small bowel obstruction due to a gallstone impacted in the distal small intestine.
2. No additional gallstones were seen, and no fistulous tract was identified.

Answers

1. Rigler triad refers to the plain film findings of pneumobilia, small bowel obstruction, and an ectopic radiopaque gallstone.
2. Surgical enterotomy with stone extraction is the standard treatment to relieve the small bowel obstruction caused by the impacted gallstone. Controversy exists in the surgical literature regarding whether the choloenteric fistula should be repaired emergently at the time of initial surgery or repaired later in the nonurgent setting.

REFERENCES

1. Lassandro F, Romano S, Ragozzino A, et al. Role of helical CT in diagnosis of gallstone ileus and related conditions. Am J Roentgenol 2005;185:1159-1165.
2. Doko M, Zovak M, Kopljar M, Glavan E, Ljubicic N, Hochstadter H. Comparison of surgical treatments of gallstone ileus: preliminary report. World J Surg 2003;27:400-404.

CLINICAL HISTORY *32-year-old woman with systemic lupus erythematosus (SLE).*

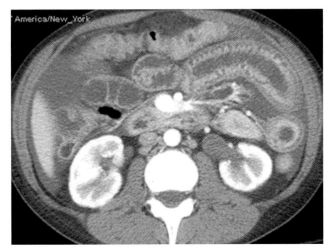

FIGURE 2.21A

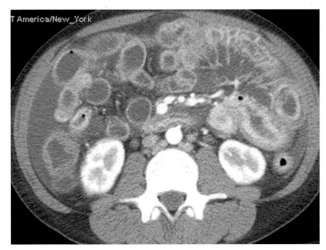

FIGURE 2.21B

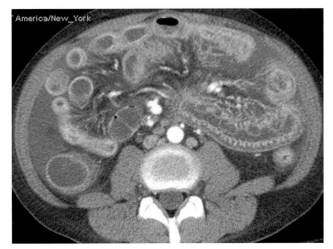

FIGURE 2.21C

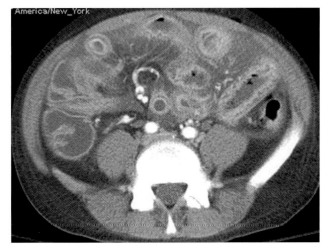

FIGURE 2.21D

FINDINGS Contrast enhanced CT images (A-D) demonstrate generalized small bowel wall thickening and luminal distention. Note the alternating levels of high and low attenuation within the bowel wall. Small volume ascites is present. There was no significant upstream bowel dilatation (not shown).

DIFFERENTIAL DIAGNOSIS Infectious enteritis, inflammatory enteritis, ischemic enteritis.

DIAGNOSIS Ischemic enteritis related to systemic lupus erythematosus (SLE).

DISCUSSION SLE is a systemic autoimmune disorder that most commonly affects women of reproductive age. A combination of genetic, environmental, and hormonal factors results in the production of immune complexes and autoantibodies that damage a variety of organs, including the brain, kidneys, and GI tract.

According to the American College of Rheumatology, at least 4 of a possible 11 criteria are necessary for a diagnosis of SLE. These criteria include malar rash, oral ulcers, arthritis, serositis, seizures, and anemia.

Small bowel manifestations of SLE include ischemia, ileus, hemorrhage, and ulceration. Intestinal ischemia results from SLE-related vasculitis. CT features of intestinal ischemia include bowel wall thickening, luminal dilatation, abnormal wall enhancement, mesenteric vascular engorgement, and ascites. The above case illustrates the double halo or target sign of intestinal ischemia which is characterized by alternating levels of low and high attenuation in the bowel wall. Patients with intestinal ischemia due to lupus usually respond to conservative management, including high-dose steroids.

Questions for Further Thought

1. How do small bowel manifestations of Henoch-Schonlein purpura (HSP) appear at CT?
2. How do small bowel manifestations of polyarteritis nodosa appear at CT?

Reporting Requirements

1. Describe the presence of a nonspecific enteritis.
2. Evaluate for evidence of bowel obstruction.

What the Treating Physician Needs to Know

1. This patient has a nonspecific enteritis.
2. No evidence of significant bowel obstruction is seen.

Answers

1. HSP is a small-vessel vasculitis that most commonly occurs in children and young adults. Frequent symptoms

in individuals with HSP are abdominal pain, arthritis, and palpable purpura. Abdominal pain may be due to intestinal ischemia, which manifests as small bowel wall thickening and mesenteric edema at CT.
2. Polyarteritis nodosa is a small- and medium-vessel vasculitis characterized by the formation of aneurysms measuring up to 1 cm in diameter. Adults in their 40s and 50s are most commonly affected by this disease. At angiography, numerous aneurysms and areas of vessel irregularity are often seen. At CT or MR, areas of ischemic bowel demonstrate bowel wall thickening, the double halo or target sign as in the above case, bowel wall dilatation, and adjacent fluid.

REFERENCES

1. Tsokos GC. Systemic lupus erythematosus. N Engl J Med 2001;365:2110-2021.
2. Byun JY, Ha HK, Yu SY, et al. CT features of systemic lupus erythematosus in patients with acute abdominal pain: emphasis on ischemic bowel disease. Radiology 1999;211:203-209.
3. Chung DJ, Park YS, Huh KC, Kim JH. Radiologic findings of gastrointestinal complications in an adult patient with Henoch-Schonlein purpura. Am J Roentgenol 2006;187:W396-W398.
4. Jee KN, Ha HK, Lee IJ, et al. Radiologic findings of abdominal polyarteritis nodosa. Am J Roentgenol 2000;174:1675-1679.

CLINICAL HISTORY *37-year-old woman with severe abdominal pain, nausea, and vomiting.*

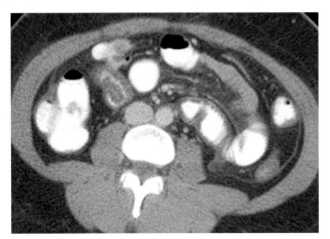

FIGURE 2.22A

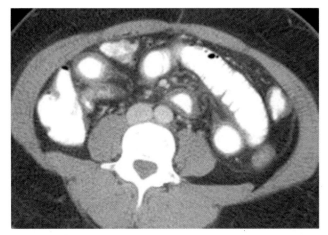

FIGURE 2.22B

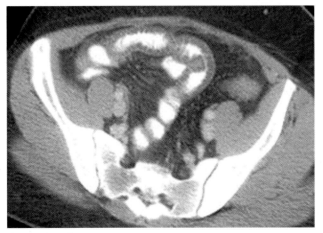

FIGURE 2.22C

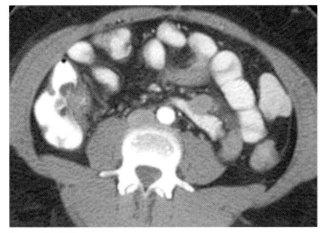

FIGURE 2.22D

FINDINGS Contrast-enhanced CT images demonstrate marked small bowel wall thickening (A) to (C). Follow-up study performed 7 days later (D) demonstrates near-complete resolution of small bowel wall thickening.

DIFFERENTIAL DIAGNOSIS Infectious enteritis, inflammatory enteritis, ischemic enteritis.

DIAGNOSIS Angiotensin-converting enzyme (ACE) inhibitor-induced angioedema of small bowel.

DISCUSSION The above initial images demonstrate nonspecific small bowel wall thickening which has a broad differential diagnosis of infection, inflammation, and ischemia. The patient was hospitalized due to the severity of her pain, and symptoms resolved over the next several days with an essentially normal appearance of small bowel at follow-up CT (D). Stool studies were negative and the etiology of the patient's symptoms remained uncertain.

The patient then developed other episodes of transient severe abdominal pain and bowel wall thickening, which again resolved during subsequent hospitalizations. During a later episode of severe abdominal pain the patient also developed a rash which was diagnosed as being related to the ACE inhibitor that the patient was taking. At this point, a correlation was noticed between severe abdominal pain that developed when the patient was an outpatient taking an ACE inhibitor with improvement in symptoms and imaging findings following hospitalization and cessation of ACE inhibitors. The patient was diagnosed with ACE inhibitor-related angioedema, was taken off ACE inhibitors, and has had no similar episodes of severe abdominal pain.

ACE inhibitor-induced small bowel angioedema often results in severe, acute abdominal pain. Development of small bowel angioedema may occur several days to several years after initiation of ACE inhibitor therapy. Symptoms usually resolve within approximately 4 days following cessation of ACE inhibitor therapy. Patients may have recurrent episodes if ACE inhibitor use continues.

CT findings include small bowel wall thickening, which can be indistinguishable from infectious, inflammatory, or ischemic enteritis. Patients often have ascites but do not demonstrate bowel obstruction.

Angioedema is thought to result from vasodilation and subsequent fluid accumulation within tissues. Angioedema may affect the tongue, throat or small bowel.

Questions for Further Thought

1. How common is ACE inhibitor-induced angioedema of any site?
2. What is nonsteroidal anti-inflammatory drug (NSAID) enteritis?

Reporting Requirements

1. Describe the presence of nonspecific bowel wall thickening.
2. Evaluate for evidence of bowel obstruction.

What the Treating Physician Needs to Know

1. The above imaging appearance is nonspecific.
2. If the patient is on ACE inhibitor therapy, the above findings could reflect ACE inhibitor-induced angioedema.

Answers

1. Angioedema is a rare complication of ACE inhibitor therapy occurring in fewer than 1% of patients with hypertension on ACE inhibitor therapy.
2. NSAIDs are another medication category that can result in small bowel pathology. Specifically, multiple circumferential short-segment small bowel strictures and small ulcerations have been described in patients with longstanding NSAID use.

REFERENCES

1. Scheirey CD, Scholz FJ, Shortsleeve MJ, Katz DS. Angiotensin-converting enzyme inhibitor-induced small-bowel angioedema: clinical and imaging findings in 20 patients. Am J Roentgenol 2011;197:393-398.
2. Vallurupalli K, Coakley KJ. MDCT features of angiotensin-converting enzyme inhibitor-induced visceral angioedema. Am J Roentgenol 2011;196:W405-W411.
3. Zalev AH, Gardiner GW, Warren RE. NSAID injury to the small intestine. Abdom Imaging 1998;23:40-44.

CLINICAL HISTORY *42-year-old woman with right lower quadrant pain and a history of renal transplant.*

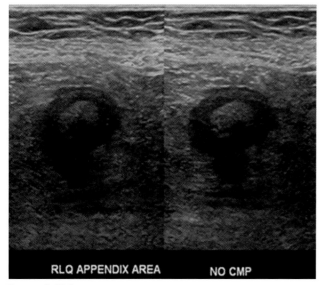

FIGURE 2.23A

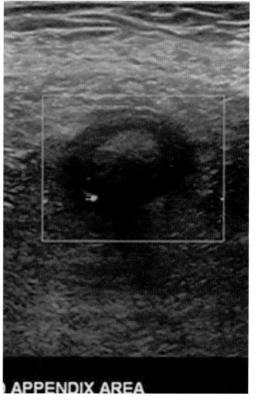

FIGURE 2.23B

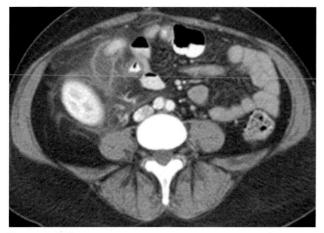

FIGURE 2.23C

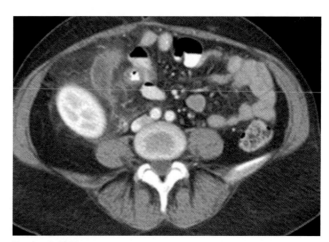

FIGURE 2.23D

FINDINGS Right lower quadrant US images obtained to evaluate the patient's renal transplant demonstrate a 2.3 cm in diameter tubular structure that is not compressible (A). Blood flow is present in the wall of this structure at color Doppler imaging (B). As this structure could not be demonstrated to be blind ending at US, the patient underwent CT for further evaluation. Contrast-enhanced CT demonstrates a thick-walled, 2.3 cm in diameter tubular structure with adjacent inflammatory changes (C, D). A 1.5-cm oval calcified intraluminal structure is present at the base of this tubular structure.

DIFFERENTIAL DIAGNOSIS Acute appendicitis, Meckel diverticulitis, terminal ileitis.

131

DIAGNOSIS   Acute appendicitis.

DISCUSSION   At US, a diagnosis of acute appendicitis can be made when a blind ending tubular structure is seen arising from the base of cecum that is not compressible and measures greater than 6 mm in diameter.

CT findings of acute appendicitis include a thick-walled appendix with periappendiceal inflammatory changes. A CT measurement "cut-off" should be used with caution when ruling in or ruling out acute appendicitis. Note that the 6-mm US "cut-off" is for appendices under direct compression. The diameter of a normal appendix at CT can vary greatly depending on whether the appendix is collapsed or the lumen is filled with fluid or air. Studies of asymptomatic patients have found that normal air-filled appendices may sometimes measure greater than 10 mm in diameter. Evaluation of appendiceal wall thickness and for periappendiceal inflammatory changes are the most helpful findings in the assessment of possible acute appendicitis at CT.

CT has been shown to be >95% sensitive and specific for the diagnosis of acute appendicitis. Potential pitfalls include mistaking an inflamed terminal ileum for acute appendicitis, but this pitfall can be avoided by confirming that the suspected appendix is indeed blind ending. Meckel diverticulitis is occasionally visible at CT and can be distinguished from acute appendicitis by noting that the Meckel diverticulum arises from the distal ileum rather than the cecal base.

Question for Further Thought

1. What findings indicate perforated appendicitis?

Reporting Requirements

1. Report that this patient has acute appendicitis.
2. Communicate this finding directly to the ordering physician.

What the Treating Physician Needs to Know

1. The patient has acute appendicitis.
2. There is no evidence of perforation.

Answer

1. Findings of perforation include extraluminal air, extraluminal appendicolith, and rim-enhancing fluid collection.

REFERENCE

1. Coursey CA, Nelson RC, Patel MB, et al. Making the diagnosis of acute appendicitis: Do more preoperative CT scans mean fewer negative appendectomies? A 10-year study. Radiology 2010;254:460-468.

CLINICAL HISTORY *72-year-old woman with several recent bloody bowel movements.*

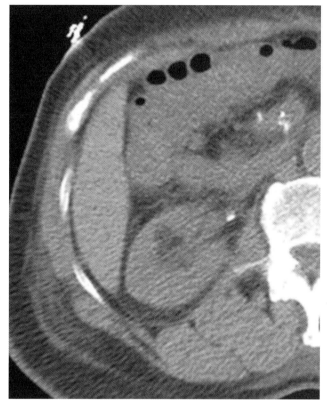

FIGURE 2.24A

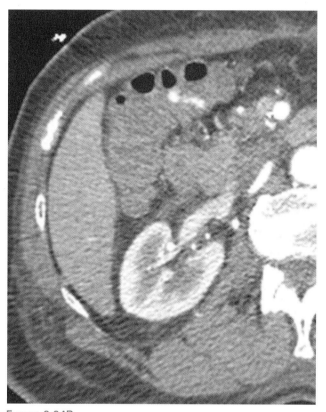

FIGURE 2.24B

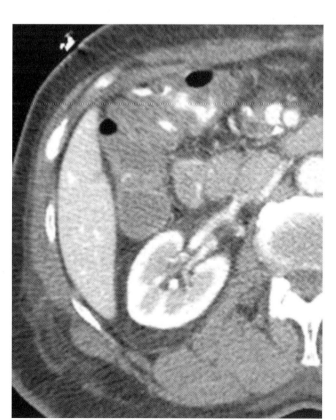

FIGURE 2.24C

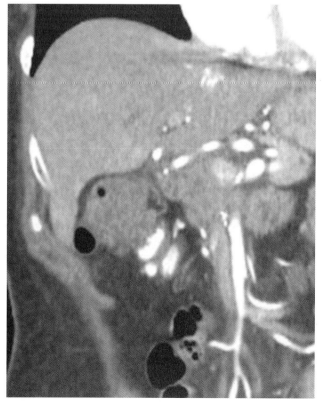

FIGURE 2.24D

FINDINGS Initial noncontrast CT image (A) demonstrates scattered vascular calcifications but no oral contrast material or any other radiopaque material in the hepatic flexure of the colon. Immediately after the noncontrast series, intravenous contrast material was administered and arterial (20 second delay) and portal venous phase (70 second delay) series were obtained. Arterial phase image (B) demonstrates an irregular accumulation of contrast material in the hepatic flexure of the colon. Portal venous phase image (C) demonstrates increased accumulation of contrast material that is as bright as the blood pool but does not conform to the expected shape of a vascular structure. Coronal reformation (D) of the arterial phase series confirms the accumulation of contrast material within the lumen of the hepatic flexure of the colon.

DIFFERENTIAL DIAGNOSIS Active bleeding, vascular malformation.

DIAGNOSIS Active bleeding.

DISCUSSION The accumulation of contrast material that is as bright as the blood pool (in other words as bright as the attenuation of the aorta) but does not conform to the expected shape of a vascular structure is diagnostic of active extravasation of contrast material which means that the patient is actively bleeding. By comparison, a vascular malformation such as an area of angiodysplasia may appear as a dilated early filling vein and a vascular tuft rather than an enlarging, ill-defined collection of contrast material.

Upper GI bleeding is defined as bleeding occurring proximal to the ligament of Treitz (esophagus, stomach, or duodenum). Lower GI bleeding is defined as bleeding that occurs distal to the ligament of Treitz (jejunum, ileum, colon, or rectum). Approximately 75% of GI bleeding originates in the upper GI tract, and the most common etiologies are ulcers and varices. The most common etiologies of lower GI track bleeding vary depending on patient age. In younger patients, inflammatory bowel disease, Meckel diverticulum, and polyps are the most common etiologies. In older patients, diverticulosis, neoplasm, and angiodysplasia are the most common etiologies.

The usual treatment algorithm for patients with GI bleeding includes esophagogastroduodenoscopy and colonoscopy to try to visualize the source of bleeding. GI bleeding sites can sometimes be treated endoscopically with banding or electrocautery.

If the site of bleeding cannot be identified endoscopically, either a technetium labeled red blood cell scan or triphasic intravenous contrast enhanced CT may be performed to try to localize the site of bleeding and serve as a road map for transcatheter embolization.

The bleeding site in the above case was supplied by a branch of the SMA. The SMA supplies inferior portions of the pancreas and duodenum (via the inferior pancreaticoduodenal artery) as well as the ileum, jejunum, and colon to the level of the mid to distal transverse colon. The remainder of the colon to the level of the upper rectum is supplied by the inferior mesenteric artery. The mid and distal rectum is supplied by branches of the internal iliac artery.

Questions for Further Thought

1. What would be an acceptable CT protocol to localize a site of GI bleeding?
2. What is the minimum bleeding rate that can be detected with a tagged red blood cell study? CT angiography? Catheter angiography?

Reporting Responsibilities

1. Describe the location of active bleeding.
2. Immediately notify the ordering physician that a bleeding site has been identified and that the patient is actively bleeding.

What the Treating Physician Needs to Know

1. The vascular territory of the bleeding site as this information will guide transcatheter embolization. In the above case, the bleeding site was arising from a branch of the SMA.

Answers

1. A triple phase protocol consisting of noncontrast, arterial, and portal venous phase images is usually performed. No positive oral contrast material should be administered as positive oral contrast material may obscure the site of GI bleeding.

   Any high attenuation material that is identified within bowel in the arterial phase images, is not present in the noncontrast images, and increases in volume in the portal venous phase images is diagnostic of a site of active bleeding. High attenuation material seen intraluminally in the postcontrast images should be compared to the noncontrast images to differentiate between extravasated contrast material and other high attenuation structures such ingested pills, suture material, or fecoliths.

2. Technetium labeled red blood cell studies can detect bleeding at rates as low as 0.1 mL per minute. Contrast enhanced CT studies can detect bleeding at rates as low

as 0.35 mL per minute. Catheter angiography can detect bleeding at rates as low as 0.5 mL per minute.

REFERENCES

1. Alavi A, Dann RW, Baum S, Biery DN. Scintigraphic detection of acute gastrointestinal bleeding. Radiology 1977;124: 753-756.

2. Hoedema RE, Luchtefeld MA. The management of lower gastrointestinal hemorrhage. Dis Colon Rectum 2005;48: 2010-2024.

3. Geffroy Y, Rodallec MH, Boulay-Coletta I, Julles M-C, Ridereaus-Zins C, Zins M, Multidetector CT angiography in acute gastrointestinal bleeding: why, when and how. Radiographics 2011;31:E35-E46.

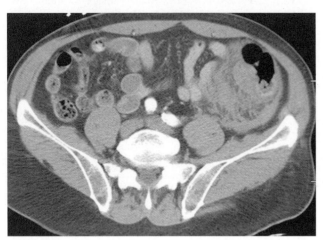

FIGURE 2.25A

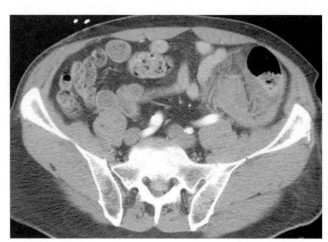

FIGURE 2.25B

FINDINGS CT images (A, B) demonstrate marked wall thickening of the sigmoid colon with high attenuation material in the adjacent mesentery.

DIFFERENTIAL DIAGNOSIS Colonic injury, mesenteric injury.

DIAGNOSIS Colonic injury with adjacent mesenteric hematoma.

DISCUSSION Bowel injuries are relatively uncommon in blunt trauma patients. However, identification of bowel injury is important as delayed diagnosis can result in significant patient morbidity due in large part to leakage of intestinal contents and abscess formation.

Bowel wall thickening with adjacent mesenteric fluid is the most sensitive finding for a significant bowel injury. The major differential diagnosis of this finding is a primary mesenteric injury with associated bowel wall thickening due to impaired venous drainage as a result of the mesenteric injury. It can sometimes be difficult to distinguish between a primary bowel injury and a primary mesenteric injury. In such cases, these patients are usually explored given the significant morbidity associated with failure to address a bowel injury.

Extraluminal orally administered contrast material is 100% specific for bowel injury but is uncommonly seen in patients with colonic injury. Pneumoperitoneum is also highly suspicious for bowel injury but can also be due to other etiologies such as barotrauma and penetrating trauma.

Question for Further Thought

1. What is the significance of a small amount of simple deep pelvic fluid in a male trauma patient without direct evidence of solid organ trauma?

Reporting Requirements

1. Describe the location of the suspected colonic injury.
2. Directly communicate this finding to the treating physician.

What the Treating Physician Needs to Know

1. That findings are highly suspicious for colonic injury.
2. The location of the injury.

Answer

1. A small volume of simple free deep pelvic fluid in male trauma patients without identifiable solid organ injury is most likely related to fluid resuscitation. A large amount of pelvic fluid in a male patient without identifiable solid organ injury could be indirect evidence of a bowel injury. A small amount of free deep pelvic simple fluid in female trauma patients of reproductive age without identifiable solid organ injury may also be physiologic.

REFERENCES

1. Brody JM, Leighton DB, Murphy BL, et al. CT of blunt trauma bowel and mesenteric injury: typical findings and pitfalls in diagnosis. Radiographics 2000;20:1525-1536.
2. Yu J, Fulcher AS, Wang D-B, et al. Frequency and importance of small amount of isolated pelvic free fluid detected with multidetector CT in male patients with blunt trauma. Radiology 2010;256:799-805.

CLINICAL HISTORY *52-year-old woman with left lower quadrant pain and urinary tract infection.*

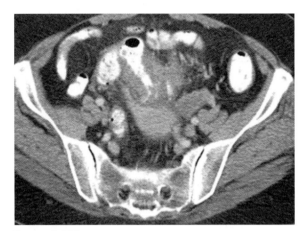

FIGURE 2.26A

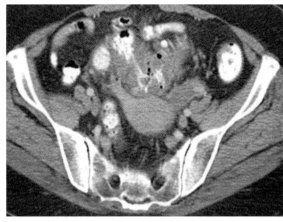

FIGURE 2.26B

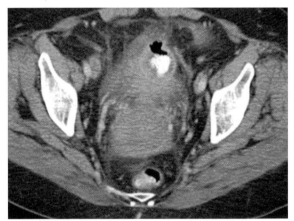

FIGURE 2.26C

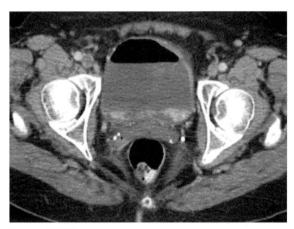

FIGURE 2.26D

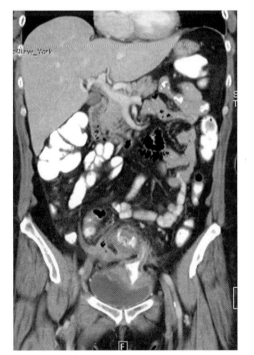

FIGURE 2.26E

FINDINGS Contrast-enhanced CT demonstrates marked segmental colonic wall thickening in an area of diverticulosis (A, B). Contrast material tracks inferiorly from this abnormal portion of the sigmoid colon to the bladder dome (C, E), which is markedly abnormally thick-walled. Orally ingested contrast material is also present within the urinary bladder (D) along with air.

DIFFERENTIAL DIAGNOSIS Uncomplicated acute diverticulitis, complicated diverticulitis.

DIAGNOSIS Complicated diverticulitis with colovesical fistula.

DISCUSSION Acute diverticulitis may be complicated by perforation, abscess formation, bowel obstruction, and fistula formation. The above case demonstrates a fistulous communication between the colon and the bladder. The presence of orally ingested contrast material in the bladder lumen is direct evidence of a fistulous communication between the bladder and the bowel.

Fistula formation is an indication for surgery. If the patient is hemodynamically stable, the operating surgeon may initially manage the patient with antibiotics to allow the inflamed colon to "cool-off". Repair of a colovesical fistula usually involves resection of the diseased portion of the colon along with bladder repair.

Question for Further Thought

1. What is the differential diagnosis of air within the lumen of the urinary bladder?

Reporting Requirement

1. Describe the presence of acute diverticulitis complicated by a colovesical fistula.

What the Treating Physician Needs to Know

1. From what segment of bowel the fistula is arising to aid in preoperative planning.
2. The portion of bladder involved by the fistula to aid in preoperative planning.

Answer

1. The differential diagnosis of air within the urinary bladder is a fistula or prior instrumentation. If the patient does not have a history of prior instrumentation (e.g., recent bladder catheter placement), a fistula should be assumed to be present until proven otherwise. Bladder fistulas most commonly arise from the colon, small intestine, or vagina.

REFERENCE

1. Jacobs DO. Clinical practice: diverticulitis. N Engl J Med 2007;357:2057-2066.

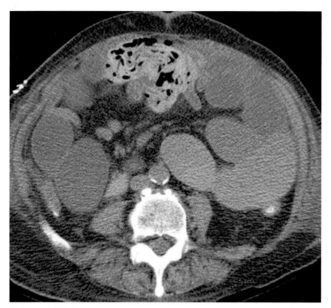

FIGURE 2.27A

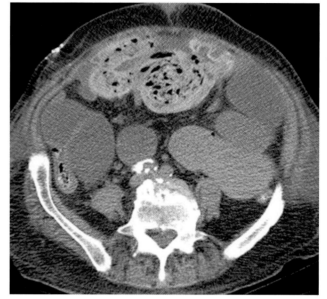

FIGURE 2.27B

FINDINGS CT images (A, B) obtained without administration of intravenous or oral contrast material demonstrate a mixed attenuation mass with areas of air in the anterior abdomen . Dilated loops of small bowel reflect a small bowel obstruction.

DIFFERENTIAL DIAGNOSIS Abscess, retained foreign body, hemostatic packing material.

DIAGNOSIS Retained foreign body (blue surgical towel), also known as a gossypiboma.

DISCUSSION The word "gossypiboma" comes from the Latin word "gossypium", which means "cotton", and the Swahili word "boma", which means "place of concealment." The term "gossypiboma" refers to retained surgical sponges, gauze, and cotton towels. Gossypibomas may become secondarily infected or may result in intestinal obstruction due to adhesions and encapsulation as in the above case.

An abscess, retained foreign body, and hemostatic packing material can all present as focal air-containing collections at CT. With an abscess, fluid is commonly seen associated with the air component. With hemostatic packing material, fluid levels are uncommon though blood products may be visible around the packing material. Correlation with recent surgical history and use of hemostatic packing material is key to avoid misdiagnosing packing material as an abscess. The thin, curvilinear areas of high attenuation visible in this case are atypical for blood products or abscess. At surgery, a blue surgical towel was found.

Questions for Further Thought

1. What is the expected imaging appearance of a gossypiboma at US?
2. What is the expected imaging appearance of a gossypiboma at MR?

Reporting Responsibilities

1. The ordering clinician should be personally notified of this unexpected finding.
2. Report the size and location of the foreign body and any complications such as bowel obstruction and secondary abscess formation.

What the Treating Physician Needs to Know

1. A foreign body is present in the abdomen.
2. The foreign body has produced a small bowel obstruction.

Answers

1. At US, a retained sponge or towel may appear as a brightly echogenic mass.
2. At MR, retained sponges and towels have varying signal intensities depending on the water component.

REFERENCES

1. Young ST, Paulson EK, McCann RL, Baker ME. Appearance of oxidized cellulose (Surgicel) on postoperative CT scans: similarity to postoperative abscess. Am J Roentgenol 1993;160:275-277.
2. Williams RG, Bragg DG, Nelson JA. Gossypiboma—the problem of the retained surgical sponge. Radiology 1978;129:323-326.

CHAPTER 3

Magnetic Resonance (MR) Imaging

CLINICAL HISTORY *65-year-old female with liver lesion noted as an incidental finding on CT performed for abdominal pain; MR obtained for further evaluation.*

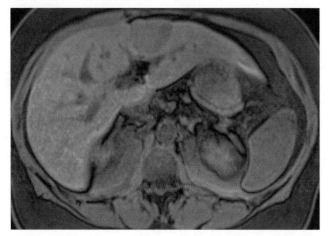

FIGURE 3.1A

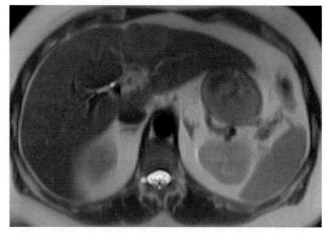

FIGURE 3.1B

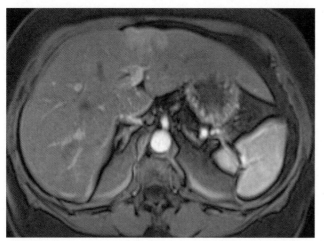

FIGURE 3.1C

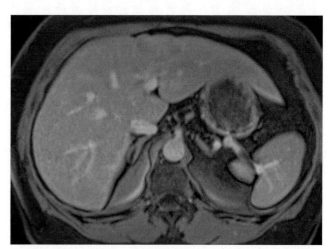

FIGURE 3.1D

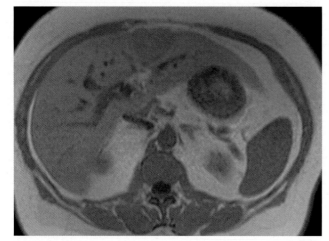

FIGURE 3.1E

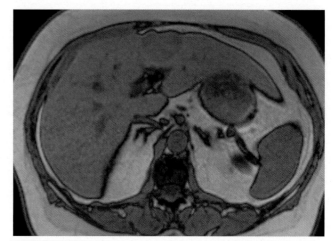

FIGURE 3.1F

FINDINGS Precontrast T1-weighted MR (A) demonstrates a 4 cm lesion in segment 4. The lesion demonstrates mildly hyperintense T2 signal (B), arterial phase hyperenhancement (C), and delayed phase washout with a capsule (D). Comparing the in-phase image (E) to the out-of-phase image (F), there are small areas of signal loss in the out-of-phase image most pronounced in the periphery of the lesion. The underlying liver parenchyma demonstrates a slightly nodular morphology.

DIFFERENTIAL DIAGNOSIS Focal nodular hyperplasia, hepatocellular adenoma, hepatocellular carcinoma.

DIAGNOSIS Hepatocellular carcinoma.

DISCUSSION The above lesion is a hyperenhancing liver lesion meaning that it enhances more avidly than the adjacent liver parenchyma in the arterial phase of enhancement (C). The lesion washes out at delayed imaging meaning that the signal in the lesion is less than that of the adjacent liver parenchyma in the delayed postcontrast image. The capsule refers to the rim of enhancement visible around the lesion in the delayed image.

Diagnostic features of a hepatocellular carcinoma are 1) hyperenhancement in the arterial phase and 2) washout with a capsule or pseudocapsule at more delayed imaging. If these requirements are met, the lesion has satisfied criteria for a hepatocellular carcinoma. Additional features of hepatocellular carcinoma that are not required for the diagnosis but are present in this case are corresponding T2 hyperintense signal and intracellular lipid as evidenced by signal loss at out-of-phase imaging.

Focal nodular hyperplasia (FNH) should not demonstrate washout with a capsule. Areas of FNH hyperenhance in the arterial phase but are stealth (imperceptible or barely perceptible) in the other phases of imaging. FNH hyperenhances at delayed phase imaging with hepatobiliary contrast agents because FNHs contain malformed biliary radicals that do not have a normal communication with the biliary system. Therefore FNHs retain hepatobiliary contrast agents longer than the adjacent hepatic parenchyma and are hyperintense at delayed imaging relative to the adjacent hepatic parenchyma with use of these contrast agents.

Hepatocellular adenomas can sometimes be difficult to distinguish from hepatocellular carcinomas. Evaluation of the background liver and patient demographics are helpful.

Morphologic changes of chronic liver disease (example, a nodular liver as in this case) favor a diagnosis of hepatocellular cancer. By comparison, a hyperenhancing lesion with intracellular lipid and washout in an otherwise healthy young woman taking oral contraceptive pills is most likely a hepatocellular adenoma.

Questions for Further Thought

1. Should this lesion be biopsied?
2. What are treatment options for this lesion?

Reporting Responsibilities

1. Describe the size and location of the hepatocellular carcinoma.
2. Notify the ordering physician of this finding.

What the Treating Physician Needs to Know

1. This patient's liver lesion is compatible with a hepatocellular carcinoma.
2. The patient has mild morphologic changes of chronic liver disease.

Answers

1. No. The lesion should not be biopsied. When a lesion is compatible with hepatocellular carcinoma based on imaging, biopsy should not be performed because of risk of tract seeding.
2. Because of her mild morphologic changes of chronic liver disease, this patient underwent a left hepatectomy. For individuals with more advanced chronic liver disease and who are within Milan criteria (up to 3 hepatocellular carcinomas ≤3 cm or 1 hepatocellular carcinoma ≤5 cm), liver transplant is the preferred treatment. Patients who are outside of Milan criteria often benefit from locoregional therapy (for example, transcatheter chemoembolization).

REFERENCES

1. Grazioli L, Morana G, Kirchin MA, Schneider G. Accurate differentiation of focal nodular hyperplasia from hepatic adenoma at gadobenate dimeglumine-enhanced MR imaging: prospective study. Radiology 2005;236:166-177.
2. Wald C, Russo MW, Heimbach JK, Hussain HK, Pomfret EA, Bruix J. New OPTN/UNOS policy for liver transplant allocation: standardization of liver imaging, diagnosis, classification, and reporting of hepatocellular carcinoma. Radiology 2013;266:376-382.

CLINICAL HISTORY *39-year-old woman presenting with right upper quadrant pain.*

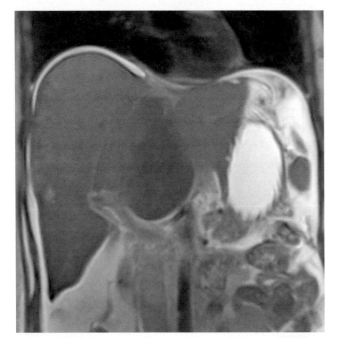

FIGURE 3.2A

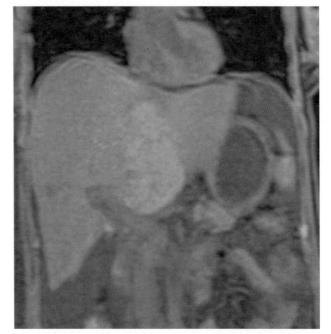

FIGURE 3.2B

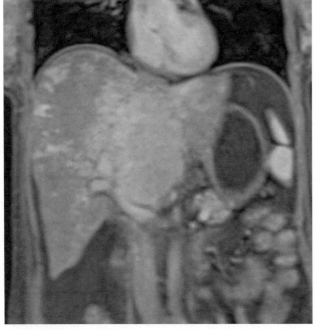

FIGURE 3.2C

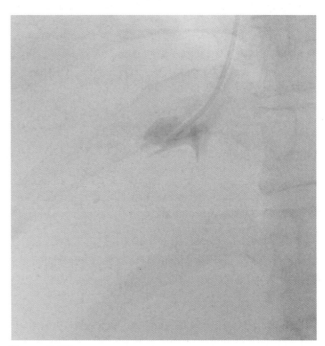

FIGURE 3.2D

FINDINGS Coronal T2-weighted (A), T1-weighted pre- (B) and postcontrast (C) images obtained through the liver. Edema is present as evidenced by increased T2 signal and decreased T1 signal with relative sparing of the caudate lobe. Postcontrast image demonstrates heterogeneous enhancement of the liver with more homogeneous enhancement of the caudate lobe (contrast agent: gadobenate dimeglumine [Gd-BOPTA, MultiHance; Bracco Diagnostics, Milan, Italy]). Venogram (D) performed via a right internal jugular vein approach demonstrates nonfilling of the central hepatic veins.

DIFFERENTIAL DIAGNOSIS Budd-Chiari syndrome, primary sclerosing cholangitis (PSC).

DIAGNOSIS Budd-Chiari syndrome.

DISCUSSION Budd-Chiari syndrome is defined as hepatic venous outflow obstruction and may be due to hypercoagulable states (e.g., antiphospholipid syndrome, protein C and S deficiencies, and pregnancy), membranous webs, or direct invasion of the hepatic veins or inferior vena cava by neoplasm (e.g., hepatocellular, adrenal, or renal cell carcinoma). Budd-Chiari syndrome most commonly occurs in women and young adults.

With acute Budd-Chiari syndrome, the liver is enlarged with heterogeneously decreased signal on T1-weighted precontrast images and increased signal on T2-weighted images indicating edema with relative sparing of the caudate lobe as in the above case. A central versus peripheral enhancement pattern also is seen with decreased and heterogeneous peripheral enhancement and relatively increased and homogeneous central enhancement. This peripheral heterogeneous enhancement occurs because of decreased blood flow due to increased tissue pressure. Relatively increased and homogeneous caudate lobe enhancement is thought to reflect alternate venous drainage of the caudate lobe.

With chronic Budd-Chiari syndrome, caudate lobe hypertrophy, irregularities of liver contour due to cirrhosis, and regenerative nodules are seen. PSC can also result in caudate lobe hypertrophy due to a separate biliary drainage pathway, but with PSC irregular intrahepatic biliary ductal dilatation is seen.

Question for Further Thought

1. What treatment options are available for Budd-Chiari syndrome?

Reporting Responsibilities

1. Identify occlusion of the hepatic veins.
2. Determine etiology of hepatic vein thrombosis (bland thrombus versus tumor thrombus).

What the Treating Physician Needs to Know

1. The extent of hepatic vein occlusion (complete versus incomplete thrombosis; are right, middle, and left hepatic veins involved?).
2. Is the thrombus bland thrombus or tumor thrombus?

Answer

1. Treatment options depend on disease severity and include medical management with anticoagulation therapy, mechanical recanalization of hepatic veins, transjugular intrahepatic portosystemic shunt (TIPS) creation, and liver transplantation. For patients with less severe disease, medical management options include managing underlying conditions, preventing further venous thrombosis with anticoagulant therapy, and management of ascites. More severe disease may necessitate attempts at hepatic vein recanalization (e.g., thrombolysis with stent placement). If attempts at recanalization fail, the patient may benefit from a TIPS or may ultimately require a liver transplant.

REFERENCES

1. Cura M, Haskal Z, Lopera J. Diagnostic and interventional radiology for Budd-Chiari syndrome. Radiographics 2009;29: 669-681.
2. Siegelman ES. Body MRI. Philadelphia, PA: Elsevier Saunders; 2005.

CLINICAL HISTORY *41-year-old woman with liver lesion seen at ultrasound performed because of elevated liver function tests. MR performed for further evaluation.*

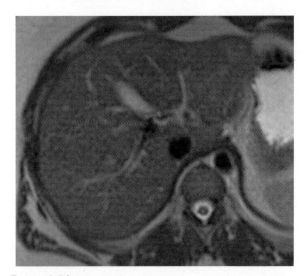

FIGURE 3.3A

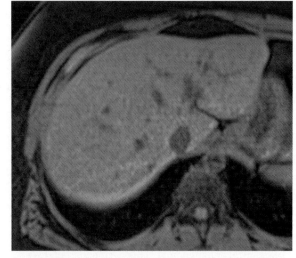

FIGURE 3.3B

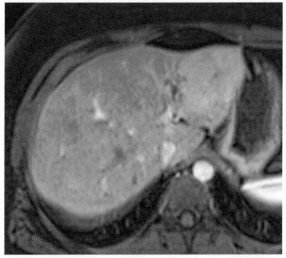

FIGURE 3.3C

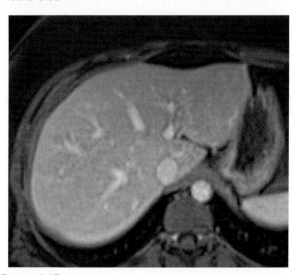

FIGURE 3.3D

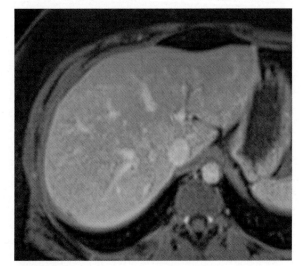

FIGURE 3.3E

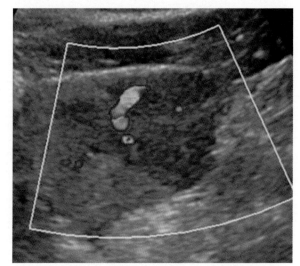

FIGURE 3.3F

FINDINGS Axial T2-weighted (A), T1-weighted precontrast (B), T1-weighted arterial phase (C), T1-weighted portal venous phase (D), and T1-weighted delayed phase (E) MR images through the upper abdomen demonstrate a 6-cm, lobulated left hepatic lobe lesion. A T2 bright central scar is visible (A). The lesion hyperenhances in the late arterial phase (C, 20-second delay), but is "stealth" or isointense to the surrounding liver parenchyma at T2-weighted (A), T1-weighted precontrast (B), venous phase (D, 70-second delay), and delayed (E, 3-minute delay) images. Delayed enhancement of the central scar is visible (E) (contrast agent: Gd-BOPTA [MultiHance; Bracco Diagnostics, Milan, Italy]). Color Doppler ultrasound image (F) demonstrates a hypoechoic mass with a central blood vessel.

DIFFERENTIAL DIAGNOSIS Focal nodular hyperplasia (FNH), hepatocellular adenoma, hepatocellular carcinoma, hemangioma, hypervascular metastasis.

DIAGNOSIS FNH.

DISCUSSION FNH is a benign hepatic tumor and is the second most common liver tumor following hemangioma. FNH is usually asymptomatic and has no malignant potential. Though the etiology of FNH is uncertain, a vascular malformation or vascular injury has been posited as the underlying event leading to the development of FNH.

At gross pathology, malformed vascular structures are visible within the central scar. Lobules of hepatic parenchyma surround the central scar and are separated by radiating fibrous bands. FNH does not have a capsule.

At MR imaging, FNH is most commonly iso- or mildly hyperintense on T2-weighted images and iso- or mildly hypointense on T1-weighted precontrast images. The central scar is frequently bright on T2-weighted images due to the presence of blood vessels, myxomatous elements, and biliary ductules. FNH avidly and homogeneously enhances in the arterial phase and becomes more isointense in the portal venous phase. The fibrous component of the central scar frequently demonstrates delayed contrast uptake. At 1- to 3-hour delayed images performed after administration of Gd-BOPTA, FNH appears iso- to hyperintense to the surrounding liver in more than 96% of cases.

At CT imaging, FNH is most commonly iso- to hypoattenuating relative to the surrounding liver at precontrast imaging, avidly and homogeneously enhances in the arterial phase, and becomes more "stealth" or isoattenuating to the surrounding liver in the portal venous phase. As with MR, the fibrous component of the central scar may demonstrate delayed contrast uptake.

Ultrasound imaging features of FNH are nonspecific. At ultrasound, FNH is usually hypoechoic and may demonstrate a central blood vessel.

Questions for Further Thought

1. How can you differentiate this tumor from hepatocellular adenoma, hemangioma, and hepatocellular carcinoma?
2. What is the usual management of FNH?

Reporting Responsibilities

1. Describe the location and size of the lesion.
2. Attempt to confidently characterize the lesion as FNH. When the diagnosis of FNH can be made with confidence at imaging, it is a "don't touch" lesion that does not warrant biopsy or surgical resection.

What the Treating Physician Needs to Know

1. Whether you are confident that the lesion is an FNH.
2. The size and location of the lesion.

Answers

1. Helpful discriminators include the above-described and illustrated enhancement pattern, absence of a capsule (both hepatocellular carcinoma and adenoma frequently demonstrate capsules), and normal background liver parenchyma (hepatocellular carcinoma most frequently occurs in cirrhotic livers). The presence of a central scar is a nonspecific finding as T2 bright central scars can be seen in hemangiomas (but hemangiomas classically demonstrate peripheral nodular enhancement with centripetal fill-in rather than homogeneous enhancement) and fibrolamellar hepatocellular carcinomas (scar is often dark on T1 and T2).
2. As these tumors have no malignant potential, they are not resected. If the diagnosis of FNH can be made with confidence at imaging, biopsy is not required.

REFERENCES

1. Hussain SM, Terkivatan T, Zondervan PE, et al. Focal nodular hyperplasia: findings at state-of-the-art MR imaging, US, CT and pathologic analysis. Radiographics 2004;24:3-17.
2. Silva AC, Evans JM, McCullough AE, et al. MR imaging of hypervascular liver masses: a review of current techniques. Radiographics 2009;29:385-402.

CLINICAL HISTORY *80-year-old man with hepatitis B and serum α-fetoprotein (AFP) level of 710 ng/mL.*

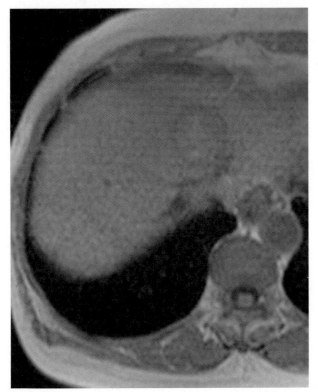

FIGURE 3.4A

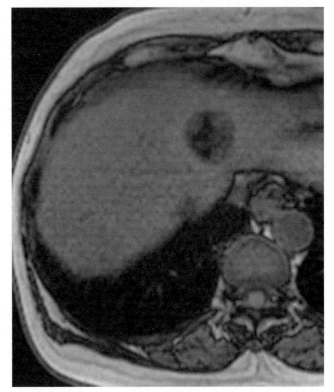

FIGURE 3.4B

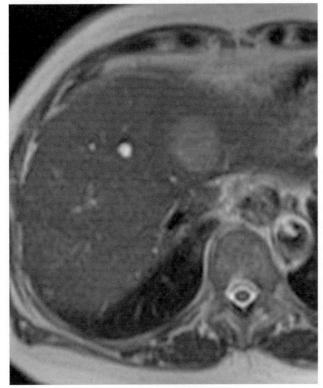

FIGURE 3.4C

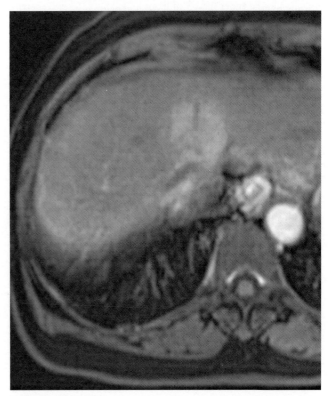

FIGURE 3.4D

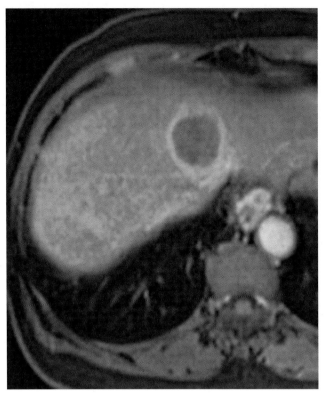

FIGURE 3.4E

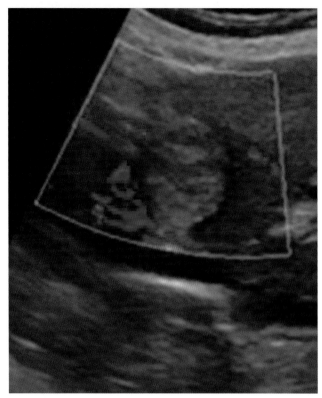

FIGURE 3.4F

FINDINGS In- (A) and out-of-phase (B) images demonstrate a 3.5-cm mass (arrows) in the segment 4a liver that loses signal in the out-of-phase images indicating that the mass contains intracellular lipid. The mass is T2 bright (C), hyperenhances in the arterial phase (D), and washes out with a capsule (E) in the delayed phase images. At color Doppler ultrasound (F), the mass is hyperechoic and heterogeneous. No discrete blood vessels could be identified in the mass at color Doppler ultrasound. This mass was new when compared with an MR imaging from 6 months prior (not shown). Incidentally noted in the T2-weighted image is a 1.2-cm T2 bright structure (C) that had imaging features compatible with a hemangioma at postcontrast imaging (not shown) (contrast agent: Gd-BOPTA [MultiHance; Bracco Diagnostics, Milan, Italy]).

DIFFERENTIAL DIAGNOSIS FNH, hemangioma, hepatocellular adenoma, hepatocellular carcinoma, metastasis from a hypervascular primary malignancy.

DIAGNOSIS Hepatocellular carcinoma.

DISCUSSION The differential diagnosis of a hyperenhancing hepatic mass is given above. Hemangioma can be eliminated from the list as the above-described mass does not demonstrate the classic peripheral discontinuous nodular enhancement with fill-in nor the T2 fluid bright signal seen with hemangiomas. FNH can be eliminated as the mass is not "stealth" in the T2-weighted image. Both hepatocellular adenoma and hepatocellular carcinoma may contain visible intracellular lipid though the patient demographics are usually quite different. Hepatic adenomas are rare tumors occurring usually in young women taking oral contraceptive pills, individuals with a glycogen storage disease, or individuals using anabolic steroids. Hepatocellular carcinomas tend to occur in patients with chronic liver disease like this patient.

Hepatocellular cancers are often bright at T2-weighted imaging. Fat-containing hepatocellular cancers will lose signal at out-of-phase imaging. About 80% to 90% of hepatocellular carcinomas are hypervascular and hyperenhancing relative to the adjacent hepatic parenchyma in the arterial phase of imaging. About 10% to 20% of hepatocellular carcinomas are relatively hypoenhancing at arterial phase imaging. Hepatocellular carcinomas demonstrate a capsule at histologic evaluation in 65% to 82% of cases, and washout with a capsule is often seen at imaging.

Questions for Further Thought

1. What conditions can result in an elevated AFP level?
2. Can the AFP level be normal in patients with hepatocellular cancer?

Reporting Responsibilities

1. Describe the size, number, and location of lesions that are compatible with hepatocellular cancer.
2. Notify the ordering clinician if the finding is unexpected.

What the Treating Physician Needs to Know

1. In patients with imaging features compatible with hepatocellular cancer (as in this case), biopsy is NOT recommended to confirm the diagnosis as biopsy may result in track seeding.
2. If the patient is suitable for liver transplant, the patient should be referred to a transplant center as liver transplant is the preferred treatment for patients with cirrhosis and hepatocellular cancer who satisfy transplant criteria (a single tumor ≤5 cm in size or not more than three tumors ≤3 cm in size).

Answers

1. A variety of tumors that can produce elevated serum AFP levels including cancers of the pancreas, stomach, and biliary tree. Liver inflammation due to chronic liver disease can also result in an elevated AFP that increases with increasing inflammation.
2. Up to 30% of patients with hepatocellular cancer may have a normal AFP at the time of diagnosis. An AFP level >400 to 500 ng/mL is thought to be diagnostic of hepatocellular cancer.

REFERENCES

1. Hanna RF, Aguirre DA, Kased N, Emery SC, Peterson MR, Sirlin CB. Cirrhosis-associated hepatocellular nodules: correlation of histopathologic and MR imaging features. Radiographics 2008;28:747-769.
2. Bialecki ED, Bisceglie AM. Diagnosis of hepatocellular cancer. HPB (Oxford) 2005;7:26-34.

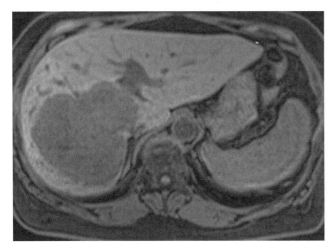

FIGURE 3.5A

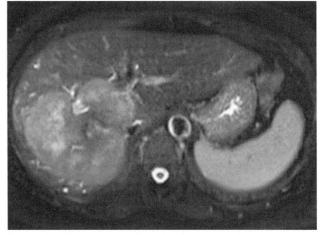

FIGURE 3.5B

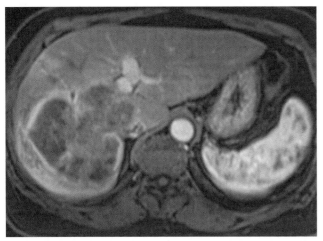

FIGURE 3.5C

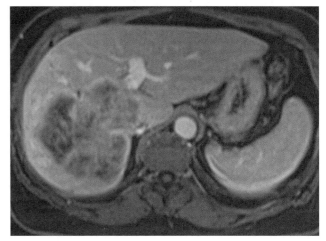

FIGURE 3.5D

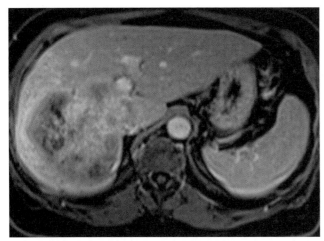

FIGURE 3.5E

FINDINGS T1- (A) and T2-weighted (B) MR images demonstrate a T1 dark mass in the right hepatic lobe with intermediate-to-bright, heterogeneous T2 signal. Postcontrast MR images in the arterial (C) and portal venous (D) phase as well as 3-minute delayed (E) MR image demonstrate progressive enhancement of the mass (contrast agent: Gd-BOPTA [MultiHance; Bracco Diagnostics, Milan, Italy]).

DIFFERENTIAL DIAGNOSIS Metastatic disease, hepatocellular carcinoma, intrahepatic cholangiocarcinoma.

DIAGNOSIS Intrahepatic cholangiocarcinoma.

DISCUSSION Cholangiocarcinoma is the second most common primary liver cancer following hepatocellular carcinoma. Cholangiocarcinomas are categorized based on location as extrahepatic, intrahepatic hilar, and intrahepatic peripheral.

At MR and CT imaging, intrahepatic cholangiocarcinomas demonstrate progressive enhancement at delayed imaging as seen in this case due to their fibrous nature. Progressive enhancement at delayed image is thought to reflect contrast material diffusing into the tumor interstitium.

By comparison, hepatocellular carcinomas classically demonstrate hyperenhancement in the arterial phase and washout at delayed imaging. An additional helpful discriminator is that cholangiocarcinomas tend to constrict adjacent vessels, whereas hepatocellular carcinomas more commonly invade adjacent vessels. Also, intrahepatic cholangiocarcinomas are often associated with more peripheral biliary ductal dilatation, whereas hepatocellular carcinomas are not. Metastatic disease could have a similar appearance to the above case, and percutaneous tissue sampling may be required to establish a diagnosis.

Questions for Further Thought

1. What are risk factors for cholangiocarcinoma?
2. What tumor markers are elevated in patients with cholangiocarcinoma?

Reporting Responsibility

1. Suggest cholangiocarcinoma in the differential diagnosis of an intrahepatic solid mass that demonstrates progressive enhancement at delayed imaging.

What the Treating Physician Needs to Know

1. Tumor size, location, and involvement of any major vascular structures.

Answers

1. Risk factors for cholangiocarcinoma include PSC, choledochal cysts, and liver fluke infestation.
2. Carcinoembryonic antigen (CEA) and carbohydrate antigen 19-9 (CA 19-9) are elevated in patients with cholangiocarcinomas but can also be elevated due to other etiologies. For example, CEA can be elevated in patients with colorectal cancer or cancers of the pancreas, lung, thyroid, or breast. CEA may also be elevated in the setting of infection and inflammatory bowel disease. CA 19-9 may also be elevated in the setting of pancreatic cancer, colorectal cancer, and gastric cancer. Nonmalignant obstructive jaundice can also result in an elevated CA 19-9.

REFERENCES

1. Han JK, Choi BI, Kim AY, et al. Cholangiocarcinoma: pictorial essay of CT and cholangiographic findings. Radiographics 2002;22:173-187.
2. Ramage JK, Donaghy A, Farrant JM, et al. Serum tumor markers for the diagnosis of cholangiocarcinoma in primary sclerosis cholangitis. Gastroenterology 1995;108:865-869.

CLINICAL HISTORY *51-year-old man with pain.*

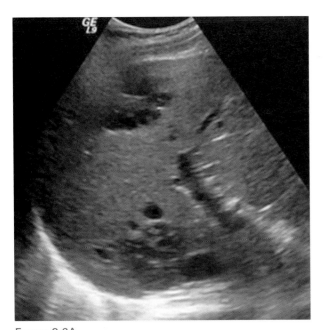

FIGURE 3.6A

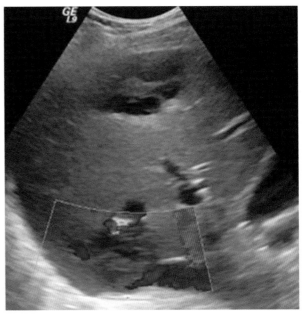

FIGURE 3.6B

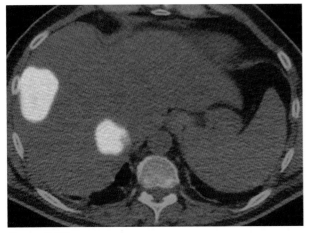

FIGURE 3.6C

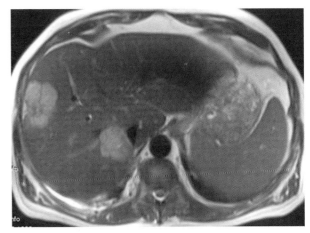

FIGURE 3.6D

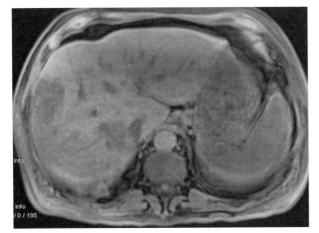

FIGURE 3.6E

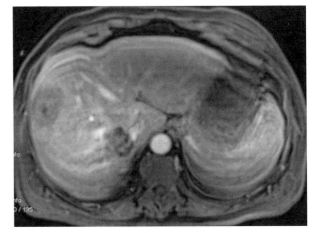

FIGURE 3.6F

FINDINGS Grayscale ultrasound image (A) demonstrates two heterogeneous, primarily hypoechoic masses in the right hepatic lobe. Color Doppler image (B) demonstrates blood flow within the posterior mass and also in the anterior mass (not shown). The masses are hypermetabolic at positron emission tomography CT imaging (C, arrows). T2-weighted MR (D) demonstrates two corresponding T2 bright areas of signal abnormality in the right hepatic lobe. The masses are dark in the T1 precontrast images (E) and hypoenhance at venous phase MR (F) (contrast agent: Gd-BOPTA [MultiHance; Bracco Diagnostics, Milan, Italy]).

DIFFERENTIAL DIAGNOSIS Abscesses, metastatic disease, lymphoma.

DIAGNOSIS Lymphoma (secondary, non-Hodgkin).

DISCUSSION Primary hepatic lymphoma is rare, accounting for less than 1% of extranodal primary lymphomas and approximately 1% of primary hepatic tumors. Primary hepatic lymphoma most commonly occurs in immunocompromised patients.

Secondary hepatic lymphoma is more common than primary hepatic lymphoma. Secondary lymphoma occurs in up to 50% of patients with non-Hodgkin lymphoma and up to 20% of patients with Hodgkin lymphoma. Secondary lymphoma is more commonly multifocal or diffusely infiltrating rather than a solitary lesion. Secondary lymphoma is usually found in patients with widespread lymphoma.

At ultrasound, hepatic lymphoma is usually hypoechoic to anechoic. At CT, hepatic lymphoma is usually hypoattenuating. At MR, hepatic lymphoma may be dark or bright on T2-weighted images, is usually dark on T1-weighted images, and is usually hypoenhancing.

Questions for Further Thought

1. What is the usual treatment for non-Hodgkin lymphoma?
2. How is the diagnosis of primary hepatic lymphoma usually made?

Reporting Responsibilities

1. Describe the size and location of the liver lesion(s).
2. Describe whether there are findings of extrahepatic disease.

What the Treating Physician Needs to Know

1. Whether the liver lesion(s) is an isolated finding or if there is other extranodal disease.
2. If the liver lesion is an isolated finding and demonstrates nonspecific imaging features, tissue sampling will likely be needed to make the diagnosis.

Answers

1. Chemotherapy is the primary treatment for non-Hodgkin lymphoma.
2. As the imaging appearance of primary hepatic lymphoma is nonspecific, tissue sampling is usually required to make the diagnosis.

REFERENCES

1. Elsayes KM, Narra VR, Yin Y, Mukundan G, Lammle M, Brown JJ. Focal hepatic lesions: diagnostic value of enhancement pattern approach with contrast-enhanced 3D gradient-echo MR imaging. Radiographics 2005;25:1299-1320.
2. Gazelle GS, Lee MJ, Hahn PF, et al. US, CT, and MRI of primary and secondary liver lymphoma. J Comput Assist Tomogr 1994;18:412-415.
3. Page RD, Romaguera JE, Osborne B, et al. Primary hepatic lymphoma: favorable outcome after combination chemotherapy. Cancer 2001;15:2023-2029.
4. Steller EJA, van Leeuwen MS, van Hillegersberg R, El Schipper M, Rinkes IHMB, Molenaar IQ. Primary lymphoma of the liver – a complex diagnosis. World J Radiol 2012;28:53-57.

CLINICAL HISTORY *45-year-old woman with abdominal pain.*

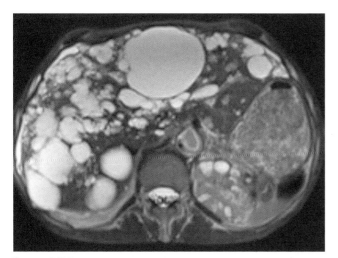

FIGURE 3.7A

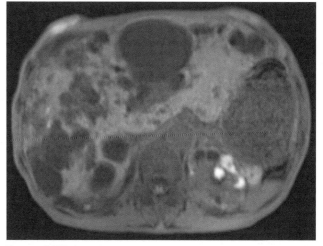

FIGURE 3.7B

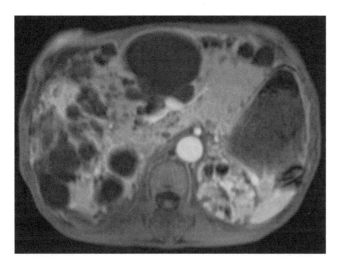

FIGURE 3.7C

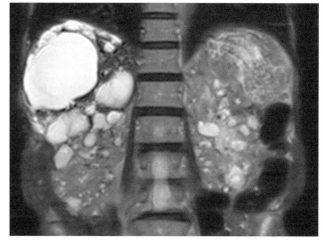

FIGURE 3.7D

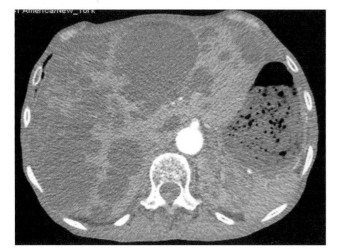

FIGURE 3.7E

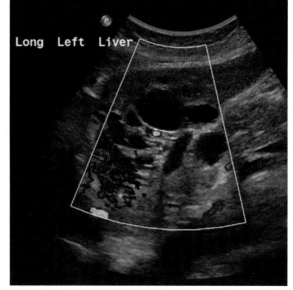

FIGURE 3.7F

FINDINGS Numerous (>20) well-circumscribed T2 bright (A) and T1 dark (B) structures are present in the liver and replace more than 50% of the hepatic parenchyma. No enhancement was seen in these structures after administration of intravenous contrast material (C). The patient also has numerous renal cysts, best seen in the coronal T2-weighted image (D). Note that some of the renal and liver lesions contain intrinsic T1 bright material reflecting small-volume blood products or proteinaceous debris (B). Numerous nonenhancing structures are also present at contrast-enhanced CT (E). Ultrasound (F) demonstrates anechoic structures with increased through transmission and no internal blood flow.

DIFFERENTIAL DIAGNOSIS Abscesses, cystic liver metastases, polycystic liver disease.

DIAGNOSIS Polycystic liver disease associated with autosomal-dominant polycystic kidney disease (ADPCKD).

DISCUSSION Polycystic liver disease most commonly occurs in association with ADPCKD but may also occur in isolation due to a separate genetic mutation that results in autosomal-dominant polycystic liver disease. Polycystic liver disease occurs in approximately 30% to 70% of patients with ADPCKD due to mutations on chromosomes 4 and 16. The genetic mutations that result in isolated polycystic liver disease have been isolated to chromosomes 6 and 19.

The cysts in polycystic liver disease are bile duct hamartomas that are lined with biliary epithelium but have no connection to the biliary system. Over time, the epithelial lining secretes fluid and the cysts progressively enlarge.

Most patients with polycystic liver disease are asymptomatic, and liver function tests are usually normal. However, a minority of patients will develop massive hepatomegaly and secondary symptoms of abdominal pain, distention, and early satiety or dyspnea due to mass effect from the massively enlarged liver. Rarely, liver cysts may hemorrhage or become infected.

At MR, the cysts associated with polycystic liver disease appear as well-circumscribed T2 bright structures. T1 signal will vary depending on cyst content. Cysts are usually dark on T1-weighted imaging but may demonstrate intrinsic T1 bright signal if they contain blood products or proteinaceous debris. If a cyst becomes infected, it may demonstrate perilesional edema and perilesional enhancement. At CT, polycystic liver disease appears as multiple well-circumscribed and nonenhancing cysts. At ultrasound, cysts associated with polycystic liver disease appear as anechoic (black) structures with increased through transmission and no internal blood flow.

Abscesses are not as homogeneous in signal intensity, may demonstrate adjacent edema, and often demonstrate abnormal enhancement such as internal septations or peripheral enhancement. Cystic liver metastases usually can be distinguished from polycystic liver disease as cystic metastases usually also have a soft-tissue component and will demonstrate areas of enhancement after administration of intravenous contrast material.

Questions for Further Thought

1. What are treatment options for patients with polycystic liver disease?
2. How many cysts are necessary for a diagnosis of polycystic liver disease?

Reporting Requirements

1. Describe the size and distribution of cysts with reference measurements of some of the larger cysts.
2. Report if the enlarged liver appears to be causing mass effect on adjacent structures such as bowel and diaphragm.
3. Report if cysts contain internal blood products or evidence of infection.

What the Treating Physician Needs to Know

1. If the patient has massive hepatomegaly with mass effect on adjacent structures.
2. If a cyst appears to contain new hemorrhage or be infected as either scenario could be a cause of patient symptoms.

Answers

1. No known medical therapy will hault cyst enlargement. Aspiration of a dominant cyst may provide brief partial symptomatic relief, but fluid within the cyst will reaccumulate. Surgical unroofing (also known as fenestration) of a cyst may be performed whereby the operating surgeon will attempt to remove as much of the cyst wall as possible. In rare cases, liver transplant may be performed for patients with severe refractory symptoms.
2. Different sources suggest different definitions of the number of cysts necessary for a diagnosis of polycystic liver disease. In general, more than 20 cysts that replace a substantial portion of the liver parenchyma should be present before a diagnosis of polycystic liver disease is invoked. Patients with fewer scattered liver cysts that occupy a small percentage of total hepatic parenchyma should not be diagnosed with polycystic liver disease based on imaging.

REFERENCES

1. Morgan DE, Lockhart ME, Canon CL, Holcombe MP, Bynon JS. Polycystic liver disease: multimodality imaging for complications and transplant evaluation. Radiographics 2006;26:1655-1668.
2. Brancatelli G, Federle MP, Vilgrain V, Vullierme M-P, Marin D, Lagalla R. Fibropolycystic liver disease: CT and MR imaging findings. Radiographics 2005;25:659-670.

3.8

CLINICAL HISTORY *38-year-old woman with hyperechoic liver lesion seen at ultrasound.*

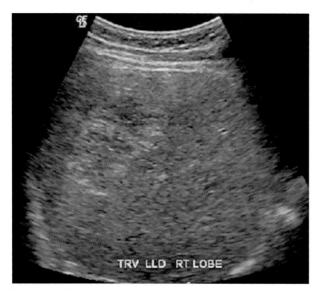

FIGURE 3.8A

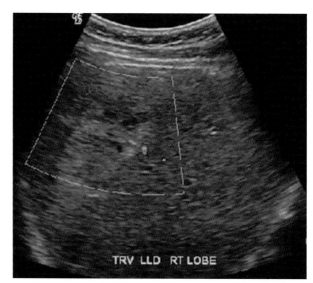

FIGURE 3.8B

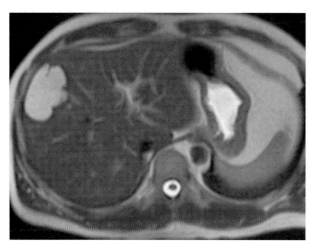

FIGURE 3.8C

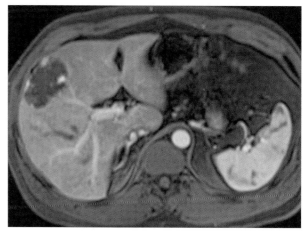

FIGURE 3.8D

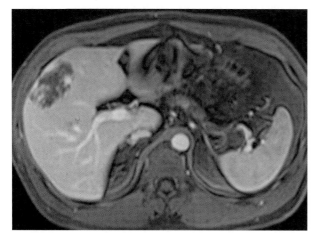

FIGURE 3.8E

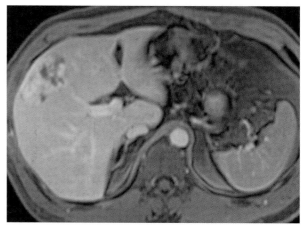

FIGURE 3.8F

FINDINGS Grayscale ultrasound (A) demonstrates an approximately 4.5-cm hyperechoic lesion in the right hepatic lobe. Color Doppler image (B) demonstrates no definite internal blood flow. Increased through transmission is seen in A and B.

T2-weighted MR demonstrates an ovoid, well-circumscribed homogeneously bright lesion in the right hepatic lobe (C). Arterial phase image (D) acquired 20 seconds after administration of intravenous contrast material demonstrates peripheral, discontinuous nodular enhancement. Venous phase image (E) acquired 70 seconds after administration of intravenous contrast material and 3-minute delayed image (F) demonstrate progressive central filling of the lesion (contrast agent: Gd-BOPTA [MultiHance; Bracco Diagnostics, Milan, Italy]).

DIFFERENTIAL DIAGNOSIS Hemangioma, hepatocellular adenoma, hepatocellular carcinoma.

DIAGNOSIS Hemangioma.

DISCUSSION Hemangiomas are common tumors occurring in up to 20% of adults and are multiple in up to 40% of patients. These tumors are usually asymptomatic and do not require treatment. In rare cases in which large hemangiomas result in discomfort or are complicated by bleeding, they may be resected.

Histologically, hemangiomas are composed of multiple vascular channels of various sizes and sparse connective tissue. Blood supply is peripheral. Blood then fills in centrally as it makes its way through these dilated vascular channels. Large hemangiomas may contain a fibrous central scar.

At contrast-enhanced cross-sectional imaging (CT or MR), classic hemangiomas demonstrate peripheral discontinuous nodular enhancement with centripetal fill-in. This peripheral nodular enhancement appears "cloud-like." The areas of peripheral nodular enhancement are often as bright as the blood pool as in the above case.

At T2-weighted MR, classic hemangiomas are homogeneously bright and may be nearly as bright as the cerebrospinal fluid (CSF). At T2-weighted imaging, hemangiomas and hepatic cysts can appear very similar but can be distinguished in postcontrast imaging based on the classic enhancement pattern of hemangiomas shown above and the absence of hepatic cyst enhancement.

At ultrasound, hemangiomas sometimes appear hyperechoic with increased through transmission and sometimes appear hypoechoic. However, malignant tumors also can appear hyperechoic at ultrasound. CT or MR should be recommended to further characterize indeterminate liver lesions identified at ultrasound. The blood flow in hemangiomas is usually too slow to be detectable at color Doppler or power Doppler ultrasound. If blood flow is detected at ultrasound, the lesion in question is most likely not a hemangioma.

Questions for Further Thought

1. What is Kasabach-Merritt syndrome?
2. What is the characteristic enhancement pattern of flash-filling hemangiomas.

Reporting Responsibilities

1. When hemangiomas demonstrate a classic appearance as above, a hemangioma can be confidently diagnosed at imaging.
2. In the setting of extremely large hemangiomas, report if there is mass effect on adjacent organs.

What the Treating Physician Needs to Know

1. Hemangiomas are benign lesions and generally require no further follow-up or treatment.
2. Hemangiomas can be confidently diagnosed at contrast-enhanced cross-sectional imaging and do not require biopsy.

Answers

1. Kasabach-Merritt syndrome is also known as hemangioma thrombocytopenia syndrome. This syndrome occurs when platelets become sequestered in a vascular tumor such as a hemangioma resulting in a consumptive coagulopathy that can ultimately progress to disseminated intravascular coagulation. Deaths have been reported. Kasabach-Merritt syndrome more commonly occurs in pediatric patients with hemangioendotheliomas but has been described in association with hemangiomas.
2. Flash-filling hemangiomas are small lesions that demonstrate marked arterial hyperenhancement in the arterial phase and are usually isointense to liver in the portal venous phase of enhancement.

REFERENCES

1. Vilanova JC, Barcelo J, Smirniotopolous JG, et al. Hemangioma from head to toe: MR imaging with pathologic correlation. Radiographics 2004;24:367-385.
2. Prasanna PM, Fredericks SE, Winn SS, Christman RA. Giant cavernous hemangioma. Radiographics 2010;30:1139-1144.

CLINICAL HISTORY *43-year-old woman with abnormal liver function tests.*

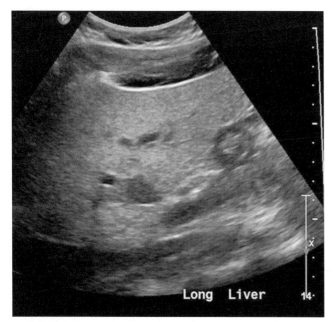

FIGURE 3.9A

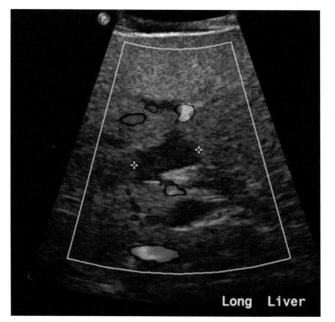

FIGURE 3.9B

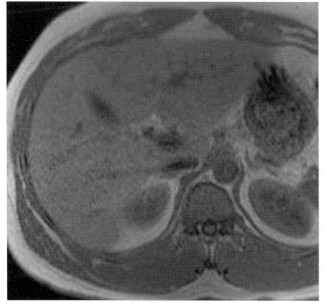

FIGURE 3.9C

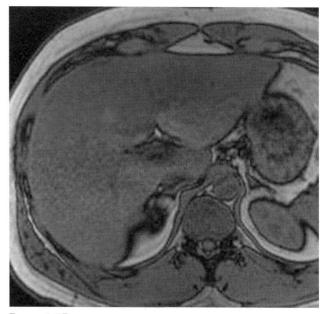

FIGURE 3.9D

FINDINGS Grayscale ultrasound (A) demonstrates an echogenic liver with a geographic hypoechoic area along the porta hepatis. No definite blood flow is visible in this area at color Doppler imaging (B, calipers). In-phase (C) and out-of-phase (D) MR demonstrate diffuse hepatic signal loss in the out-of-phase image with the exception of the hepatic parenchyma around the porta hepatis.

DIFFERENTIAL DIAGNOSIS Hepatic steatosis with fat sparing; hepatic steatosis with focal fat deposition.

DIAGNOSIS Hepatic steatosis with fat sparing.

DISCUSSION Histologically, fatty liver is characterized by the accumulation of triglycerides within hepatocyte cells. At

159

ultrasound, hepatic steatosis is characterized by increased echogenicity of the liver (liver brighter than kidney) and loss of definition of anatomy within the liver. Fat sparing appears as a geographic relatively hypoechoic area.

At MR, signal loss at out-of-phase imaging indicates the presence of fat. That the area around the porta hepatis demonstrates relatively brighter signal in the out-of-phase image indicates that there is fat sparing in this location. Typical areas of focal fat sparing or deposition include around the porta hepatis, gallbladder fossa, falciform ligament, and elsewhere in the subcapsular liver. It has been postulated that variant venous drainage in these locations contributes to preferential fat deposition or sparing in these areas.

Focal fat deposition or sparing sometimes can be difficult to distinguish from true liver lesions. Clues to the presence of focal fat deposition or sparing include the following: a characteristic location, geographic morphology rather than round shape, nondistorted vessels extending through the area, and enhancement less than or equal to adjacent normal liver.

Nonalcoholic fatty liver disease is a generic term encompassing both fatty liver and non-alcoholic steatohepatitis (NASH). NASH refers to liver inflammation secondary to accumulation of fat in the liver. NASH can progress to chronic liver disease/cirrhosis and is now a leading cause of liver disease leading to transplantation at some centers.

Questions for Further Thought

1. List conditions associated with NASH.
2. How can you identify the out-of-phase image?

Reporting Requirements

1. This patient has diffuse hepatic steatosis.
2. The geographic hypoechoic area seen at ultrasound reflects an area of fat sparing.

What the Treating Physician Needs to Know

1. Further evaluation to determine the etiology of hepatic steatosis is warranted.
2. If untreated, steatosis can progress to steatohepatitis and ultimately hepatic fibrosis.

Answers

1. Obesity, type 2 diabetes, high cholesterol, elevated triglycerides, and metabolic syndrome are associated with NASH.
2. The out-of-phase images can be identified by noting the "India ink artifact" (also known as chemical shift artifact of the second kind). The India ink artifact describes the solid black line at all fat–water interfaces that looks as if it were drawn with India ink.

REFERENCE

1. Hamer OW, Aguirre DA, Casola G, Lavine JE, Woenckhaus M, Sirlin CB. Fatty liver: imaging patterns and pitfalls. Radiographics 2006;26:1637-1653.

CLINICAL HISTORY *53-year-old man with chronic liver disease undergoing screening for hepatocellular cancer.*

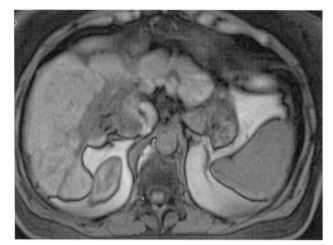

FIGURE 3.10A

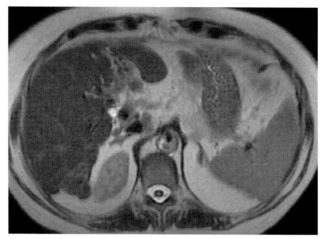

FIGURE 3.10B

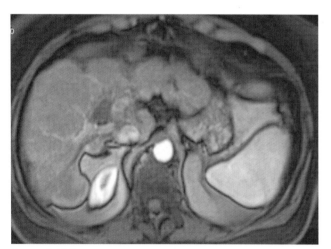

FIGURE 3.10C

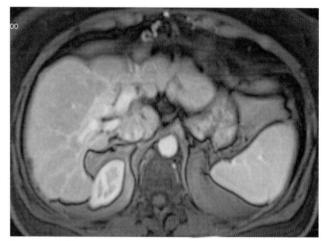

FIGURE 3.10D

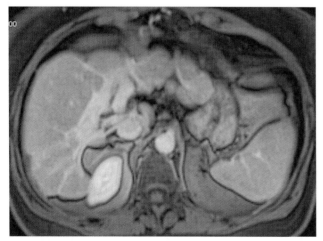

FIGURE 3.10E

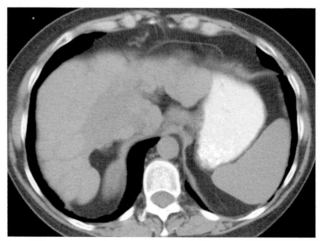

FIGURE 3.10F

FINDINGS T1-weighted MR (A) demonstrates a small, nodular liver in keeping with changes of advanced chronic liver disease. Notice also the geographic area of low signal with linear margins involving primarily segments 4A and 8 near the inferior vena cava. T2-weighted MR demonstrates corresponding T2 bright signal abnormality in segments 4A (B) and 8 (not shown). Dynamic contrast-enhanced MR demonstrates this area to be hypoenhancing relative to adjacent hepatic parenchyma in the arterial phase (C) of enhancement, hyperenhancing in the portal venous phase (D), and extremely hyperenhancing in the 3-minute delayed image (E) (contrast agent: Gd-BOPTA [MultiHance; Bracco Diagnostics, Milan, Italy]). Noncontrast CT (F) demonstrates a corresponding area of low attenuation.

DIFFERENTIAL DIAGNOSIS Confluent hepatic fibrosis.

DIAGNOSIS Confluent hepatic fibrosis.

DISCUSSION Hepatic fibrosis occurs in response to liver injury such as chronic inflammation due to hepatitis. Liver fibrosis is histologically defined as the deposition of substances including collagen and proteoglycans in the extracellular matrix.

The phrase "confluent fibrosis" refers to large, mass-like areas of fibrosis. Confluent fibrosis most commonly involves the anterior segment right hepatic lobe and medial segment left hepatic lobe.

At MR, areas of fibrosis usually demonstrate low T1 signal and high T2 signal due to the presence of water within areas of fibrosis. Areas of fibrosis exhibit delayed hyperenhancement at both CT and MR due to accumulation of gadolinium in the extracellular compartment. Areas of fibrosis can be thought of as hanging on to contrast material while contrast material washes out from the remainder of the liver. Delayed hyperenhancement in areas of confluent hepatic fibrosis is usually relatively homogeneous.

Confluent hepatic fibrosis can be distinguished from a neoplasm by its geographic morphology often with linear borders, associated capsular retraction, relatively homogeneous delayed hyperenhancement, and progressive volume loss over time.

Questions for Further Thought

1. What intrahepatic malignancy contains fibrous tissue and may demonstrate delayed hyperenhancement?
2. List other fibrotic conditions elsewhere in the body that demonstrate delayed hyperenhancement.

Reporting Requirements

1. Describe the presence of confluent hepatic fibrosis.
2. Describe any sequelae of portal hypertension such as splenomegaly, varices, and ascites.
3. Careful attention should be paid to evaluate for hepatocellular cancer in patients with findings of chronic liver disease.

What the Treating Physician Needs to Know

1. That the patient has areas of confluent hepatic fibrosis.
2. If the patient has findings of portal hypertension or evidence of hepatocellular cancer.

Answers

1. Intrahepatic cholangiocarcinomas often demonstrate delayed hyperenhancement at contrast-enhanced MR due to the presence of fibrous tissue. Intrahepatic cholangiocarcinomas can be distinguished from areas of confluent fibrosis based on morphology. For example, intrahepatic cholangiocarcinomas usually have infiltrating or rounded borders, whereas confluent hepatic fibrosis is frequently geographic in shape with linear borders. Though intrahepatic cholangiocarcinomas often show delayed hyperenhancement, the enhancement is more heterogeneous than is seen with confluent hepatic fibrosis. Additionally, intrahepatic cholangiocarcinomas are often associated with biliary ductal dilatation more peripherally, whereas areas of confluent hepatic fibrosis are not.
2. Retroperitoneal fibrosis and mesenteric fibrosis can also demonstrate delayed hyperenhancement due to the presence of fibrous tissue.

REFERENCES

1. Fein SC, Ganesan K, Mwangi I, et al. MR imaging of liver fibrosis: current state of the art. Radiographics 2009;29:1615-1635.
2. Elsayes KM, Narra VR, Yin Y, Mukundan G, Lammle M, Brown JJ. Focal hepatic lesions: diagnostic value of enhancement pattern approach with contrast-enhanced 3D gradient-echo MR imaging. Radiographics 2005;25:1299-1320.

CLINICAL HISTORY *68-year-old man with abnormal liver function tests 3 months after liver transplant.*

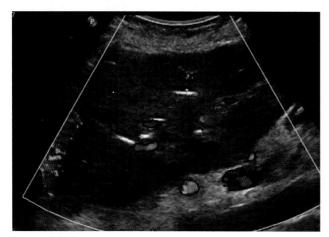

FIGURE 3.11A

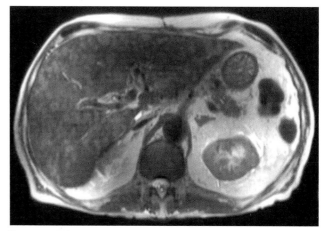

FIGURE 3.11B

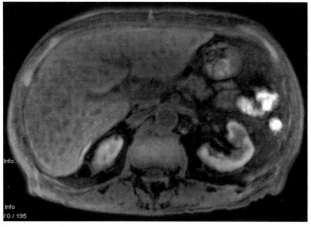

FIGURE 3.11C

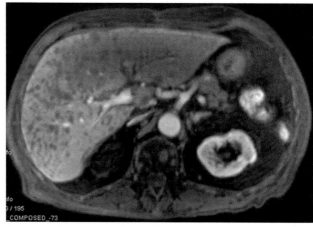

FIGURE 3.11D

FINDINGS Color Doppler ultrasound demonstrates heterogeneous hepatic parenchyma (A) and patent transplant vasculature (not shown). Patient next underwent MR imaging to better evaluate the liver parenchyma. T2-weighted MR (B) demonstrates innumerable 1- to 2-cm T2 bright liver lesions that are T1 dark (C) and hypoenhancing (D) (contrast agent: Gd-BOPTA [MultiHance; Bracco Diagnostics, Milan, Italy]).

DIFFERENTIAL DIAGNOSIS Abscesses, post-transplant lymphoproliferative disorder (PTLD), metastatic disease.

DIAGNOSIS PTLD.

DISCUSSION PTLD occurs as a complication of organ transplantation due to immunosuppression. A majority of cases appear to be related to Epstein-Barr virus. PTLD is a general term that describes a spectrum of illnesses. At the milder end of the spectrum, some patients will manifest an acute mononucleosis-type illness. At the more severe end of the spectrum, patients develop a monoclonal proliferation of lymphoid cells that meet diagnostic criteria for lymphoma. Liver biopsy was performed in the above patient, and pathology revealed B-cell lymphoma.

PTLD is uncommon occurring in approximately 1% to 2% of liver transplant patients. PTLD is slightly more common in other solid organ transplant patients (e.g., kidney and lung) and occurs in up to a third of patients who undergo bowel transplant or multiple organ transplants.

Of patients who develop PTLD, a majority of patients will develop PTLD in the first year after transplant when immunosuppression is most intense. At imaging, patients with PTLD may present with solid organ lesions or lymphadenopathy with extranodal disease being more common. PTLD preferentially involves the transplanted organ. Central nervous system and gastrointestinal tract involvement also may occur. The mainstay of treatment of PTLD is cessation or decrease in immunosuppressive medications.

Abscesses could have a similar appearance at imaging, though fever and elevated white blood cell count would be expected. Diffuse metastatic disease could have a similar appearance. Tissue sampling is usually required to make the diagnosis of PTLD.

Questions for Further Thought

1. What is the typical clinical presentation of PTLD?
2. What are the most common locations of gastrointestinal involvement with PTLD?

Reporting Requirement

1. If solid organ lesions or marked lymphadenopathy are seen in a transplant recipient, suggest the possibility of PTLD.

What the Treating Physician Needs to Know

1. Solid organ lesions or lymphadenopathy could reflect PTLD in a transplant recipient.
2. Tissue sampling will likely be needed to confirm the diagnosis.

Answers

1. Clinical presentation of PTLD can be quite variable. Many patients are initially asymptomatic. However, given the propensity of PTLD to involve the transplanted organ or the gastrointestinal tract, evidence of graft dysfunction or diarrhea could reflect PTLD.
2. Distal small bowel and proximal colon are the most commonly affected bowel segments. PTLD appears similar to nontransplant-related lymphoma and may manifest as segmental bowel wall thickening with aneurysmal dilatation.

REFERENCES

1. Borhani AA, Hosseinzadeh K, Almusa O, Furlan A, Nalesnik M. Imaging of posttransplantation lymphoproliferative disorder after solid organ transplantation. Radiographics 2009;29: 981-1000.
2. Shanbhogue AKP, Virmani V, Vikram R, et al. Spectrum of medication-induced complications in the abdomen: role of cross-sectional imaging. Am J Roentgenol 2011;197: W286-W294.

CASE 3.12

CLINICAL HISTORY *67-year-old woman with right upper quadrant pain.*

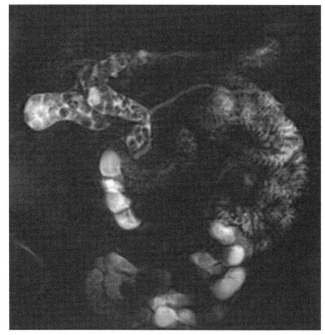

FIGURE 3.12A

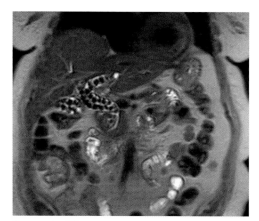

FIGURE 3.12B

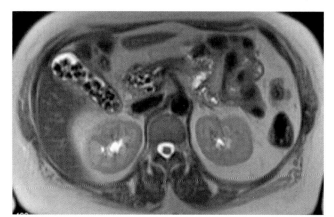

FIGURE 3.12C

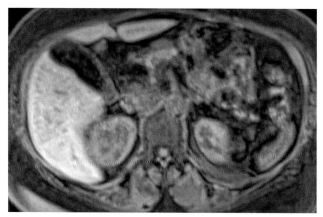

FIGURE 3.12D

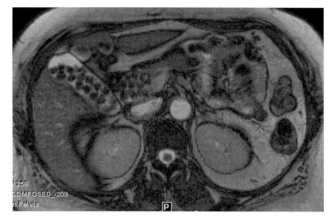

FIGURE 3.12E

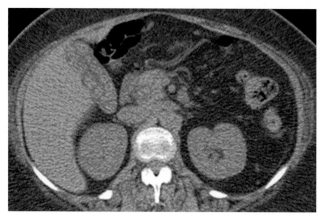

FIGURE 3.12F

FINDINGS Slab image from MRCP (A) demonstrates innumerable T2 dark-filling defects within the gallbladder, central intrahepatic biliary ducts, and in the extrahepatic bile duct. These filling defects are confirmed in the coronal (B) and axial T2-weighted images (C) and demonstrate low signal in the T1 precontrast (D) and True FISP images (E). At CT, these structures appear as well-circumscribed areas of increased attenuation (F).

DIFFERENTIAL DIAGNOSIS Air bubbles, gallstones, flow voids.

DIAGNOSIS Gallstones.

DISCUSSION The differential diagnosis of multiple areas of low T2 signal within the biliary system includes air bubbles, gallstones, and flow voids. The rounded shape and dependent location of the above intraluminal structures are diagnostic of gallstones.

Gallstones may contain cholesterol, glycoproteins, and/or calcium bilirubinate. All stones usually appear dark at T2-weighted imaging. Cholesterol stones also appear dark at T1-weighted imaging, whereas pigment stones appear bright at T1-weighted imaging.

A way to evaluate for the presence of air in the biliary system is to compare signal intensity with in- and out-of-phase images. Air will "bloom" or appear darker and larger in the in-phase images if in-phase images are obtained with a longer TE. The reason for this finding is that air produces magnetic susceptibility artifact, and this artifact increases with longer TE.

A way to distinguish flow voids from gallstones is to look at the True FISP images. True FISP images are relatively insensitive to motion. Flow voids are usually not visible at True FISP imaging. Therefore, if focal low signal is visible within the biliary system on the True FISP images it is most likely a gallstone.

MRCP is a heavily T2-weighted MR technique whereby fluid-containing structures demonstrate high signal (appear bright). Note in the above case how fluid in the biliary system and pancreatic duct is bright. Note also the bright fluid in the lumen of the duodenum located just inferior to the biliary system. Fluid is also visible within jejunal loops in the left abdomen as well as ileal loops in the right lower quadrant.

Question for Further Thought

1. How sensitive are radiographs, ultrasound, CT, and MR for the detection of gallstones?

Reporting Requirements

1. Report the presence of innumerable stones filling the gallbladder and biliary system.
2. Evaluate for complications such as cholecystitis or pancreatitis.

What the Treating Physician Needs to Know

1. This patient has innumerable gallstones filling the biliary system.
2. There is no evidence of acute cholecystitis or pancreatitis.

Answer

1. Abdominal radiographs are approximately 15% to 20% sensitive for the detection of gallstones. Ultrasound is 95% sensitive for the detection of gallstones larger than 2 mm in size. CT is 75% sensitive for the detection of gallstones and is better able to detect calcium-containing stones when compared with cholesterol-containing stones. MR is >95% sensitive for the detection of gallstones.

REFERENCES

1. Catalano OA, Sahani DV, Kalva SP, et al. MR imaging of the gallbladder: a pictorial essay. Radiographics 2008;28:135-155.
2. Grand D, Horton KM, Fishman E. CT of the gallbladder: spectrum of disease. Am J Roentgenol 2004;183:163-170.

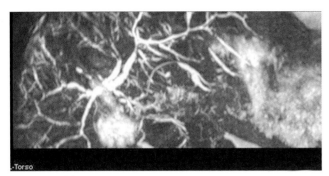

FIGURE 3.13A

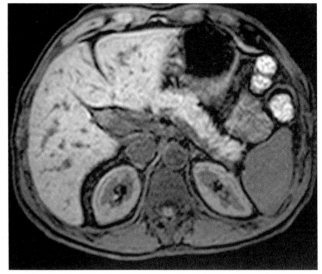

FIGURE 3.13B

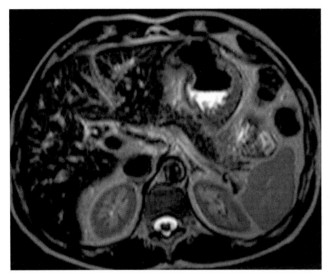

FIGURE 3.13C

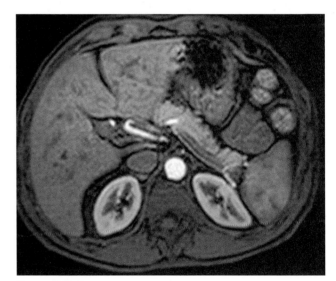

FIGURE 3.13D

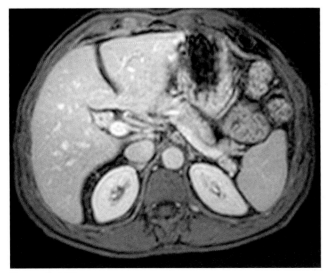

FIGURE 3.13E

FINDINGS MRCP slab image (A) demonstrates mild-to-moderate intrahepatic biliary ductal dilatation with abrupt termination just beyond the confluence of the right and left hepatic ducts. Note also the irregularity of the intrahepatic biliary system with areas of relative dilatation and stricturing.

Axial T1 MR (B) demonstrates circumferential low signal surrounding the extrahepatic bile duct just below the confluence of the right and left hepatic ducts. Corresponding T2 dark signal is present surrounding the T2 bright bile duct (C).

Postcontrast images demonstrate this material to be hypoenhancing in the arterial phase (D) and relatively hyperenhancing in the 3-minute delayed images (E). Note that this mass-like area is located along the right posterior aspect of the right hepatic artery (D) and along the right aspect of the main portal vein (E).

DIFFERENTIAL DIAGNOSIS Stricture, cholangiocarcinoma.

DIAGNOSIS Cholangiocarcinoma.

DISCUSSION When measurable soft tissue is present at the site of abrupt bile duct termination or tapering as in the above case, cholangiocarcinoma is present until proven otherwise. Cholangiocarcinomas may be intrahepatic, perihilar, or extrahepatic in location. Perihilar is the most common location as in the above case.

The Bismuth classification is used to characterize perihilar cholangiocarcinomas. Type 1 tumors involve the common hepatic duct below the confluence of the right and left hepatic ducts. Type 2 tumors involve the confluence of the right and left hepatic ducts. Type 3a tumors are type 2 tumors that also extend to the bifurcation of the right hepatic duct. Type 3b tumors are type 2 tumors that extend to the bifurcation of the left hepatic duct. Type 4 tumors extend to the bifurcation of the right and left hepatic ducts. Type 5 tumors are located at the junction of the common bile duct and the cystic duct.

The above case was characterized as a Bismuth 2 lesion. The irregularity of the intrahepatic biliary system visible in the slab MRCP image reflects the patient's underlying diagnosis of primary sclerosis cholangitis, a risk factor for cholangiocarcinoma.

Historically, surgical resection has been the treatment of choice for cholangiocarcinomas. The relationship of the tumor to major vascular structures such as the hepatic artery and portal vein strongly influences surgical decisions regarding resectability. More recently, liver transplants are being performed at some centers to treat hilar cholangiocarcinomas with positive outcomes.

Questions for Further Thought

1. What are Klatskin tumors?
2. How could tissue sampling be performed in the above case?

Reporting Requirements

1. Describe the presence of a hilar soft-tissue mass resulting in intrahepatic biliary ductal dilatation.
2. Describe the relationship of the mass to major vascular structures such as the hepatic artery and portal vein.
3. Evaluate for distant metastatic disease such as liver metastases.

What the Treating Physician Needs to Know

1. This patient has an obstructing hilar cholangiocarcinoma on a background of PSC.
2. The tumor abuts the right hepatic artery and the main portal vein.
3. No distant metastatic disease is visible.

Answers

1. Klatskin tumors are cholangiocarcinomas that occur at the confluence of the right and left hepatic ducts. Gerald Klatskin (1910 to 1986) was an American pathologist and hepatologist.
2. Tissue sampling could be performed via brushings with endoscopic retrograde cholangiopancreatography (ERCP). Brushings can also be performed during transhepatic cholangiopancreatography.

REFERENCES

1. Sainani NI, Catalano OA, Holalkere N-S, Zhu AX, Hahn PF, Sahani DV. Cholangiocarcinoma: current and novel imaging techniques. Radiology 2008;28:1263-1287.
2. Kanne JP, Rohrmann CA Jr, Lichtenstein JE. Eponyms in radiology of the digestive tract: historical perspectives and imaging appearances. Part 2. Liver, biliary system, pancreas, peritoneum, and systemic diseases. Radiographics 2006;26:465-480.

CLINICAL HISTORY *53-year-old woman 3 years status post-liver transplant now with pruritus and elevated bilirubin.*

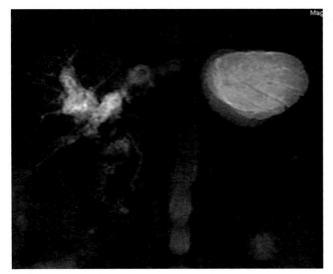

FIGURE 3.14A

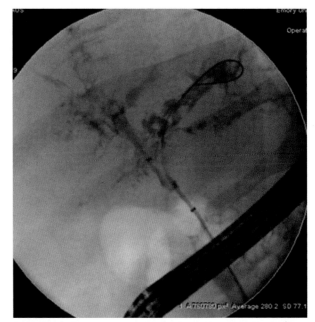

FIGURE 3.14B

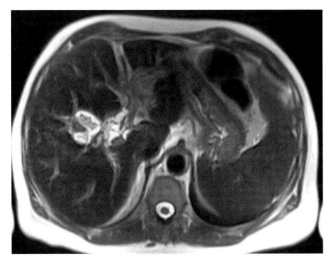

FIGURE 3.14C

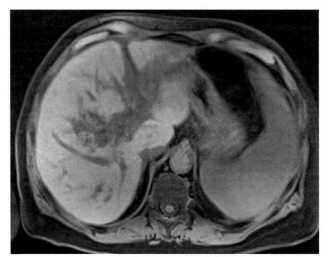

FIGURE 3.14D

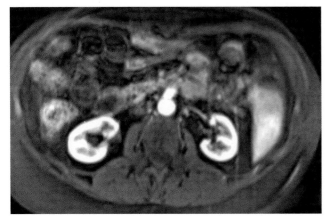

FIGURE 3.14E

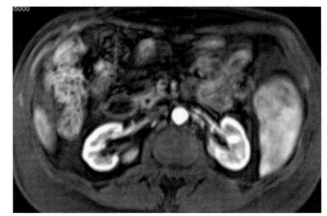

FIGURE 3.14F

FINDINGS Slab MRCP (A) demonstrates severe intrahepatic biliary ductal dilatation with peripheral pruning of the biliary tree. Multiple filling defects are identified within the intrahepatic biliary system. The common bile duct is decompressed. ERCP (B) performed for stent placement confirms marked irregularity of the intrahepatic biliary system with numerous rounded filling defects. These filling defects are dark at T2-weighted MR (C) and bright at T1-weighted MR (D). Arterial phase postcontrast images demonstrate the hepatic artery jump graft to be patent at its aortic origin (E). The graft occludes just beyond its origin (F).

DIFFERENTIAL DIAGNOSIS Anastomotic stricture, ischemic cholangiopathy.

DIAGNOSIS Ischemic cholangiopathy; also intraductal stones and sludge due to stasis.

DISCUSSION Biliary ductal irregularity and stricturing with an occluded hepatic artery or hepatic artery jump graft is diagnostic of ischemic cholangiopathy. The hepatic artery provides the sole blood supply to the biliary system of the transplanted liver. Hepatic artery occlusion consequently results in bile duct ischemia, necrosis, and eventual stricturing.

Biliary complications are the second most common cause of liver transplant failure and occur in approximately 15% of liver transplant recipients. When evaluating a post-liver transplant patient at ultrasound or cross-sectional imaging, it is critically important to evaluate the patency of the hepatic artery, portal vein, and hepatic veins. Failure to identify and address an occluded hepatic artery can result in ischemic cholangiopathy that may necessitate retransplantation.

Question for Further Thought

1. What is another potential biliary complication of liver transplant?

Reporting Requirements

1. Describe the presence of bile duct stricturing and dilatation.
2. Evaluate the patency of the hepatic artery

What the Treating Physician Needs to Know

1. This patient has ischemic cholangiopathy due to an occluded arterial jump graft.

Answer

1. Bile duct leak is a potential acute complication of liver transplant. Chronically, liver transplant patients may also develop focal strictures at the biliary anastomosis. Anastomotic strictures are often due to localized ischemia or scarring rather than proximal hepatic arterial occlusion.

REFERENCES

1. Novellas S, Caramella T, Fournol M, Gugenheim J, Chevallier P. MR cholangiopancreatography features of the biliary tree after liver transplantation. Am J Roentgenol 2008;191:221-227.
2. Ostroff JW. Management of biliary complications in the liver transplant patient. Gastroenterol Hepatol 2010;6:264-272.

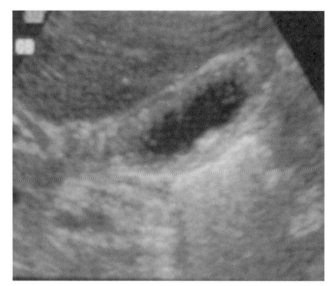

FIGURE 3.15A

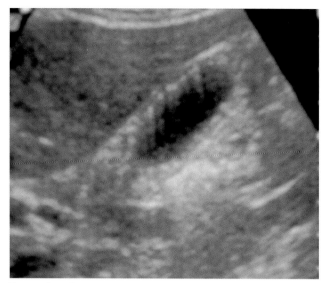

FIGURE 3.15B

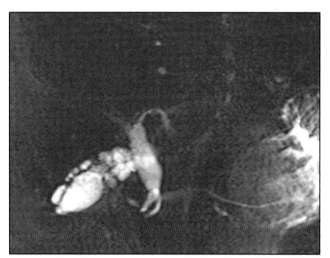

FIGURE 3.15C

Adenomyomatosis is characterized by gallbladder wall thickening, intramural diverticula, and deposition of cholesterol crystals in these diverticula. Fluid-filled diverticula correspond to the cystic spaces seen at MR. When multiple cystic spaces are visible in the gallbladder wall as in the above case, the appearance has been referred to as the "pearl necklace sign."

The comet tail artifact seen at ultrasound is reverberation artifact seen posterior to cholesterol crystals in Rokitansky-Aschoff sinuses and is characterized by multiple parallel echogenic bands posterior to an object.

Adenomyomatosis may be diffuse, segmental, or focal. Segmental adenomyomatosis most commonly occurs in the gallbladder body and results in wasting with an hourglass appearance. Focal adenomyomatosis most commonly occurs at the gallbladder fundus. Focal or segmental adenomyomatosis can sometimes be difficult to distinguish from gallbladder cancer at ultrasound. If MR is not definitive, fluorine 18 fluorodeoxyglucose positron emission tomography can be used to distinguish the two entities as gallbladder cancer will appear hypermetabolic while focal adenomyomatosis will not.

FINDINGS Grayscale ultrasound images (A, B) demonstrate diffuse gallbladder wall thickening. Note the echogenic material with parallel bands of increased echogenicity posteriorly ("comet tail" artifact). Note the area of cystic change in the gallbladder wall as seen at MRCP (C).

DIFFERENTIAL DIAGNOSIS Adenomyomatosis, emphysematous cholecystitis.

DIAGNOSIS Adenomyomatosis.

DISCUSSION The comet tail artifact seen at ultrasound and cystic spaces seen in the gallbladder wall at MRCP are characteristics of adenomyomatosis.

Questions for Further Thought

1. What is cholesterolosis?
2. What symptoms may be associated with adenomyomatosis?
3. What is the usual treatment of adenomyomatosis?

Reporting Requirements

1. Describe the presence of diffuse adenomyomatosis.

What the Treating Physician Needs to Know

1. Adenomyomatosis alone is usually not considered an indication for cholecystectomy.

Answers

1. Though the terms "adenomyomatosis" and "cholesterolosis" are sometimes used interchangeably, technically these terms refer to two different and distinct conditions. Adenomyomatosis refers to deposition of cholesterol crystals within Rokitansky-Aschoff sinuses in the gallbladder wall with corresponding wall thickening seen at ultrasound. By comparison, cholesterolosis refers to cholesterol crystal deposition along the lamina propria of the gallbladder and is usually not associated with gallbladder wall thickening.

2. Patients with adenomyomatosis may be asymptomatic or have vague abdominal pain.

3. Adenomyomatosis is thought to have no malignant potential and therefore requires no further treatment.

REFERENCES

1. Boscak AR, Al-Hawary M, Ramsburgh SR. Adenomyomatosis of the gallbladder. Radiographics 2006;26:941-946.

2. Shapiro RS, Winsberg F. Comet-tail artifact from cholesterol crystals: observations in the postlithotripsy gallbladder and an in vitro model. Radiology 1990;177:153-156.

CASE 3.16

CLINICAL HISTORY *62-year-old woman with vague right upper quadrant pain.*

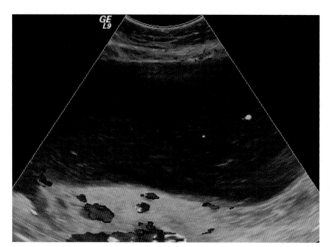

FIGURE 3.16A

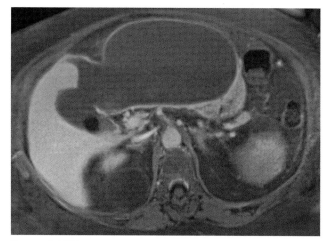

FIGURE 3.16B

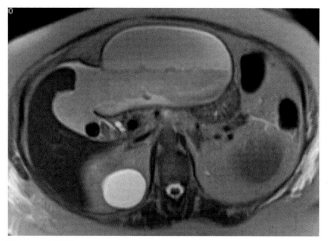

FIGURE 3.16C

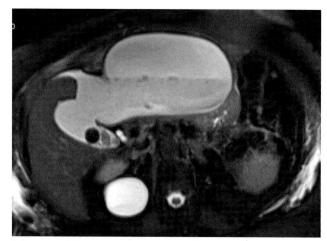

FIGURE 3.16D

FINDINGS Color Doppler ultrasound (A) demonstrates a 20-cm well-circumscribed hypoechoic structure with layering debris but no definite internal blood flow. T1-weighted MR image obtained 60 seconds after administration of intravenous contrast material (B) demonstrates rim enhancement around the area of fluid. Note that fluid is contiguous with the gallbladder lumen through an approximately 3-cm gallbladder wall defect. A 1-cm T1 dark stone is present in the gallbladder lumen. T2-weighted MR without (C) and with (D) fat saturation demonstrate primarily T2 bright fluid with layering-dependent relatively lower signal debris. Note also T2 dark gallstone. (Incidentally noted 3.5-cm cyst exophytic off the upper pole right kidney.)

DIFFERENTIAL DIAGNOSIS Perforated acute cholecystitis, remote prior gallbladder perforation.

DIAGNOSIS Contained remote prior gallbladder perforation.

DISCUSSION T2-weighted images with fat saturation are crucial when assessing for the presence or absence of acute inflammation. Acute inflammation is indicated by T2 bright signal reflecting fluid. Such signal is much more conspicuous against a background of dark fat in T2-weighted images obtained with fat saturation. The absence of T2 bright inflammatory changes around the above fluid collection in the T2 with fat saturation image indicates that the abnormality is chronic rather than acute.

The above patient had a history of acute cholecystitis approximately 6 weeks prior to the above study and was pain free at the time of the above study. The patient underwent percutaneous drainage of the above fluid collection and later underwent elective cholecystectomy.

Gallbladder perforation is thought to result when intraluminal pressure increases due to outflow obstruction. This increased intraluminal pressure results in impaired blood flow, tissue necrosis, and eventual tissue breakdown.

Question for Further Thought

1. What portion of the gallbladder most commonly perforates?

Reporting Requirements

1. Describe the presence of a large fluid collection contiguous with the gallbladder lumen.
2. Assess for acute inflammatory changes.

What the Treating Physician Needs to Know

1. This patient has a large fluid collection likely reflecting a remote prior gallbladder perforation.
2. No significant acute inflammatory changes are visible about the collection.

Answer

1. The gallbladder fundus is the most common site of perforation, possibly due to a tenuous blood supply in this location.

REFERENCE

1. Morris BS, Balpande PR, Morani AC, Chaudhary RK, Maheshwari M, Raut AA. The CT appearance of gallbladder perforation. Br J Radiol 2007;80:898-901.

CLINICAL HISTORY *26-year-old woman with history of abdominal pain.*

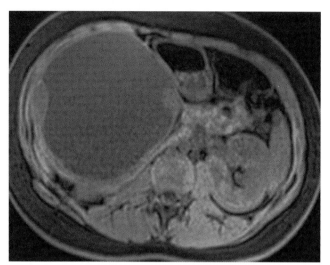

FIGURE 3.17A

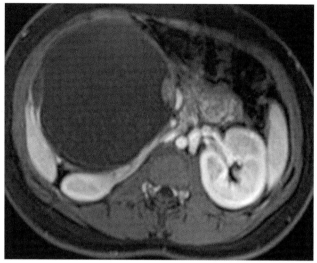

FIGURE 3.17B

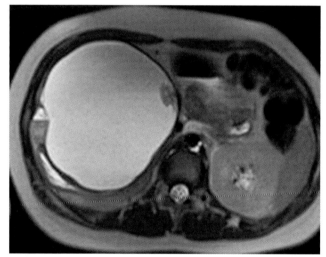

FIGURE 3.17C

FINDINGS MR image demonstrates a 15-cm primarily cystic mass with small, peripheral solid components in the region of the pancreatic head. The cystic components demonstrate T1 dark signal (A) and T2 bright signal (C). The peripheral solid components enhance at postcontrast imaging (B). No enlarged lymph nodes or distant metastatic disease were seen.

DIFFERENTIAL DIAGNOSIS Pancreatic adenocarcinoma, neuroendocrine tumor, acinar cell carcinoma, solid pseudo-papillary tumor (SPT).

DIAGNOSIS SPT of the pancreas.

DISCUSSION SPT of the pancreas is a rare neoplasm that accounts for 1% to 2% of pancreatic exocrine malignancies. These tumors most commonly occur in non-Caucasian women in the second or third decade of life.

SPTs most frequently occur in the pancreatic head or tail and appear as large well-circumscribed cystic masses with peripheral solid components as in the above case. However, when small these tumors may appear entirely solid.

These tumors usually exhibit benign behavior. However, since up to 15% of SPTs undergo malignant degeneration all tumors thought to be SPTs are usually resected.

The tumor gets its name from its distinct appearance at microscopy where cells are arranged in solid and papillary configurations.

The well-circumscribed nature of SPTs distinguishes them from the more ill-defined, infiltrating appearance typical of pancreatic ductal adenocarcinomas. The imaging appearance of SPTs can be similar to acinar cell carcinomas as acinar cell tumors are also well-circumscribed tumors that may appear solid when small and contain large cystic components when large. However, SPTs most commonly occur in young women, whereas pancreatic acinar carcinomas most commonly occur in patients in the fifth through seventh decades of life. Small SPTs can be difficult to distinguish from neuro-endocrine tumors. The peripheral papillary solid projections seen in large primarily cystic SPTs is atypical for neuroendocrine tumors.

Questions for Further Thought

1. What lab abnormalities are associated with SPT?
2. What is the usual treatment for SPT?

Reporting Responsibilities

1. Describe the size and location of the mass.
2. Evaluate for nodal or other metastatic disease.

What the Treating Physician Needs to Know

1. That an SPT is favored rather than a ductal adenocarcinoma as this information may alter treatment planning (see Question 2).

Answers

1. None. Pancreatic cancer markers (CA19-9, AFP, CEA) are normal in patients with SPT.

2. Surgical resection is usually curative. At the present time, there is no roll for neoadjuvant chemotherapy in these patients. By comparison, neoadjuvant chemotherapy may be administered to patients with pancreatic ductal adenocarcinomas. Therefore, tissue sampling may be performed prior to resection to determine if neoadjuvant chemotherapy is warranted in questionable cases.

REFERENCES

1. Coleman K, Doherty MC, Bigler SA. Solid-pseudopapillary tumor of the pancreas. Radiographics 2003;23: 1644-1648.
2. Cantisani V, Mortele KJ, Levy A, et al. MR imaging features of solid pseudopapillary tumor of the pancreas in adult and pediatric patients. Am J Roentgenol 2003;181:395-401.

CLINICAL HISTORY *44-year-old woman with abdominal pain.*

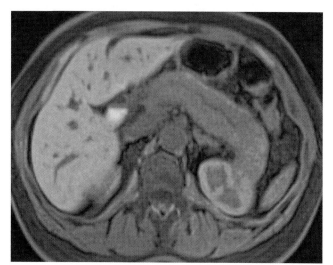

FIGURE 3.18A

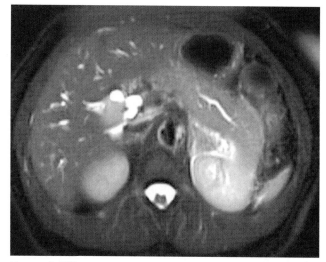

FIGURE 3.18B

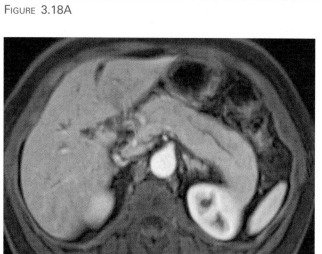

FIGURE 3.18C

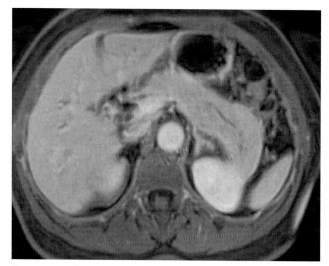

FIGURE 3.18D

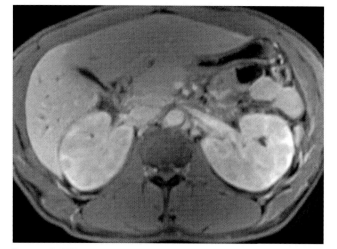

FIGURE 3.18E

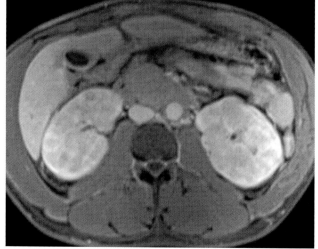

FIGURE 3.18F

FINDINGS T1 precontrast MR (A) demonstrates diffuse enlargement of the pancreas and loss of expected T1 bright signal. A thin T2 bright peripancreatic halo is visible (B). This halo demonstrates hyperenhancement at arterial (C) and delayed phase (D) imaging. Note also innumerable ill-defined patchy areas of hypoenhancement in the renal parenchyma of a different patient with the same diagnosis (E, F).

DIFFERENTIAL DIAGNOSIS Alcohol-related pancreatitis, autoimmune pancreatitis, gallstone pancreatitis.

DIAGNOSIS Autoimmune pancreatitis.

DISCUSSION Autoimmune pancreatitis is a manifestation of IgG4 sclerosing disease and is characterized by plasma cell infiltration of the pancreas, often with associated inflammation and fibrotic change.

At imaging, autoimmune pancreatitis appears as diffuse enlargement of the pancreas or as focal or multifocal masses. The diffuse form may appear similar to acute pancreatitis, whereas the focal form can mimic pancreatic adenocarcinoma.

In the diffuse form of autoimmune pancreatitis, the pancreas is diffusely enlarged. A thin rim or halo of low attenuation is visible at CT. At MR, a thin halo of T2 bright signal is present and often demonstrates delayed hyperenhancement indicating fibrous tissue. By comparison, patients with acute pancreatitis often exhibit more ill-defined and a larger amount of peripancreatic inflammation.

Focal autoimmune pancreatitis most commonly occurs in the pancreatic head or uncinate process and can manifest as an isoattenuating or hypoattenuating mass that can be difficult to distinguish from pancreatic adenocarcinoma. Patients with autoimmune pancreatitis or pancreatic adenocarcinoma resulting in biliary ductal dilatation may both present with painless jaundice. Biopsy may be necessary to distinguish between these two entities.

IgG4 sclerosing disease can also involve a variety of other structures including the biliary system, kidneys, and retroperitoneum. Specifically, segmental biliary strictures may be visible along with hypoenhancing areas in the kidneys (E, F) and retroperitoneal fibrosis. Though not present in every case, identification of these other findings can help in distinguishing focal autoimmune pancreatitis from pancreatic adenocarcinoma.

Questions for Further Thought

1. What laboratory abnormalities may be present in patients with autoimmune pancreatitis?
2. What is the usual treatment of autoimmune pancreatitis?

Reporting Requirements

1. Report that the appearance of the pancreas is most suggestive of autoimmune pancreatitis.
2. Evaluate for involvement of other organs such as hypoenhancing renal lesions and biliary strictures.

What the Treating Physician Needs to Know

1. This patient most likely has autoimmune pancreatitis.

Answers

1. Patients with autoimmune pancreatitis often have elevated IgG4 antibody levels. However, some patients with pancreatic adenocarcinoma may also have elevated IgG4 antibody levels.
2. Patients with autoimmune pancreatitis are usually treated with steroids. A pancreatic mass due to autoimmune pancreatitis would be expected to decrease in size during the course of steroid treatment.

REFERENCES

1. Sahani DV, Kalva SP, Farrell J, et al. Autoimmune pancreatitis: imaging features. Radiology 2004;233:345-352.
2. Vlachou PA, Khalili K, Jang H-J, Fischer S, Hirschfield GM, Kim TK. IgG4-related sclerosing disease: autoimmune pancreatitis and extrapancreatic manifestations. Radiographics 2011;31:1379-1402.

CLINICAL HISTORY *31-year-old pregnant woman with right lower quadrant pain.*

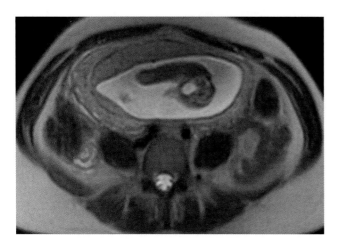

FIGURE 3.19A

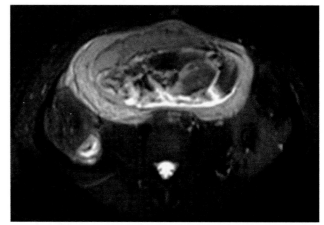

FIGURE 3.19B

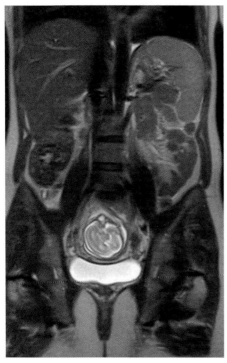

FIGURE 3.19C

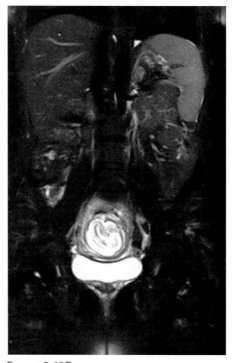

FIGURE 3.19D

FINDINGS Axial (A) and coronal (C) T2-weighted MR demonstrate the appendix located in the right lower quadrant arising from the base of cecum. Axial (B) and coronal (D) T2-weighted MR with fat saturation demonstrate marked T2 bright signal surrounding the appendix.

DIFFERENTIAL DIAGNOSIS Normal appendix, acute appendicitis.

DIAGNOSIS Acute appendicitis.

DISCUSSION Noncontrast MR is the preferred modality to evaluate for acute appendicitis in pregnant women. MR is preferred over CT because MR does not expose the fetus to ionizing radiation. Contrast material should not be administered to pregnant women as gadolinium-based contrast agents are excreted into the amniotic fluid thereby subjecting the fetus to prolonged exposure.

A satisfactory MR protocol to evaluate for acute appendicitis in pregnant women includes coronal, sagittal, and axial

T2-weighted images; coronal and axial T2-weighted images with fat saturation; axial True FISP images; axial in- and out-of-phase images; and axial and coronal T1-weighted images.

Multiplanar T2-weighted images are used to identify the appendix. T2-weighted images with fat saturation are key to evaluate for periappendiceal inflammation. The periappendiceal inflammation visible in the above case (B, D) is diagnostic of acute appendicitis. Without fat saturation (A, C), bright signal indicating fluid and inflammation can be difficult or impossible to identify on a background of T2 bright fat. Note how periappendiceal inflammation is much more obvious in the T2-weighted images with fat saturation (B, D) when compared with the T2-weighted images without fat saturation (A, C).

True FISP images serve as a backup sequence to identify the appendix as True FISP images are often the least sensitive to motion. T1-weighted images are most helpful to evaluate for other causes of right lower quadrant pain such as a hemorrhagic cyst that would contain T1 bright material. In- and out-of-phase images can be used to evaluate for extraluminal air which would be expected to "bloom" (appear darker and larger) in the in-phase images with longer TE due to increased susceptibility artifacts with longer TE.

As with CT, findings of perforation at MR include periappendiceal fluid collections and extraluminal air.

Question for Further Thought

1. Are there any risks to a fetus undergoing MR imaging?

Reporting Requirements

1. Report that the patient has acute appendicitis.
2. Report whether or not the patient has evidence of perforation.

What the Treating Physician Needs to Know

1. This patient has acute appendicitis.
2. There are no findings to indicate perforation.

Answer

1. The major risk of noncontrast MR is heat deposition in the fetus. No current literature indicates that this minimal heat deposition has deleterious effects on the fetus. The risks of performing MR in a pregnant patient should always be weighed against the potential benefit of the study and the potential risk of not performing the study. In general, the benefits of performing noncontrast MR to evaluate for acute appendicitis are thought to outweigh the risks at all stages of pregnancy.

REFERENCE

1. Spalluto LB, Woodfield CA, DeBenedectis CM, Lazarus E. MR imaging evaluation of abdominal pain during pregnancy: appendicitis and other nonobstetric causes. Radiographics 2012;32:317-334.

CLINICAL HISTORY *51-year-old man with generalized abdominal pain.*

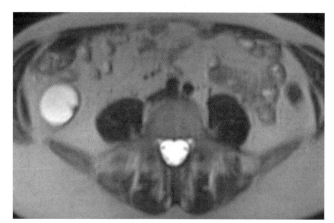

FIGURE 3.20A

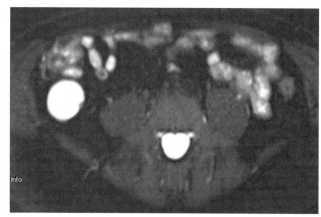

FIGURE 3.20B

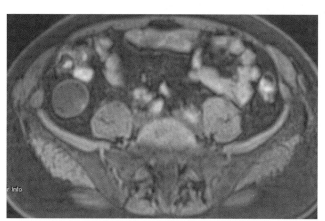

FIGURE 3.20C

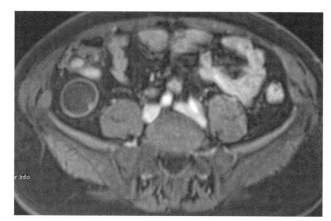

FIGURE 3.20D

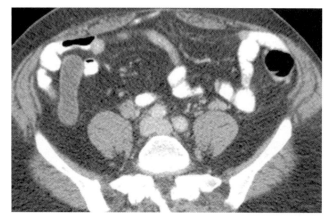

FIGURE 3.20E

FINDINGS T2-weighted MR without (A) and with (B) fat saturation demonstrate a 2.7 cm in diameter T2 bright structure in the right lower quadrant. This structure was determined to be arising from the base of cecum in other images of the study. Pre- (C) and postcontrast (D) MR images demonstrate a small 3-mm-enhancing nodule along the medial wall of the structure. This enhancing nodule demonstrates low signal in the T2-weighted images (A, B). CT image from a different patient (E) with the same diagnosis demonstrates a distended appendix filled with low-attenuation material and no surrounding inflammatory changes.

DIFFERENTIAL DIAGNOSIS Normal fluid-containing appendix, appendiceal mucocele.

DIAGNOSIS Appendiceal mucocele due to mucinous cystadenoma.

DISCUSSION Appendiceal mucocele is defined as an appendix distended with mucin. At CT, mucoceles appear as homogeneous low-attenuation material distending the appendix. Periappendiceal inflammatory changes usually are absent. At MR, mucoceles generally demonstrate homogeneously bright T2 signal. T1 signal will vary depending on whether appendiceal contents are mostly fluid (T1 dark) or whether blood products or proteinaceous debris are present (T1 bright signal).

Mucin may accumulate in the appendix due to outflow obstruction or due to a mucin-producing tumor such as a benign cystadenoma or a malignant cystadenocarcinoma. Both cystadenomas and cystadenocarcinomas can perforate resulting in mucinous material filling the abdomen and pelvis, a condition known as pseudomyxoma peritonei.

The enhancing small nodule in the above MR images is somewhat unusual as most often no enhancing solid component is seen. If an enhancing solid component is visible, the patient has a cystadenoma or cystadenocarcinoma.

Question for Further Thought

1. What is the usual management of an appendiceal mucocele?

Reporting Requirements

1. Report the presence of an appendiceal mucocele.
2. Report that the small soft-tissue nodule most likely indicates a cystadenoma or cystadenocarcinoma.

What the Treating Physician Needs to Know

1. This patient has an appendiceal mucocele most likely due to a cystadenoma or cystadenocarcinoma.

Answer

1. Appendiceal mucoceles are virtually always removed due to the risk of malignant transformation. If no soft-tissue component is visible, the mucocele will likely be removed via appendectomy. If there is suspicion for malignancy, a right hemicolectomy will be performed with removal of regional lymph nodes.

REFERENCE

1. Honnef I, Moschopulos M, Roeren T. Appendiceal mucinous cystadenoma. Radiographics 2008;28:1524-1527.

3.21

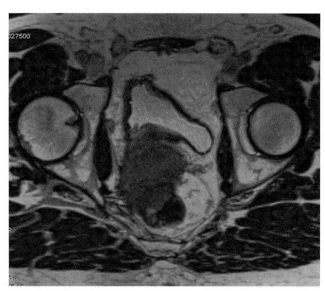

FIGURE 3.21

FINDINGS High-resolution T2-weighted MR image through the pelvis demonstrates rectal wall thickening extending from approximately 7 o'clock to 1 o'clock. The mass extends beyond the serosal surface of the rectum as well as the mesorectal fascia from approximately 9 o'clock to 1 o'clock. Tumor invades the right posterior bladder wall.

DIFFERENTIAL DIAGNOSIS T1–T4 rectal cancer.

DIAGNOSIS T4 rectal cancer.

DISCUSSION T staging of known rectal cancer is an increasingly common indication for MR imaging. T1 disease is defined as tumor that invades the submucosa. T2 disease invades the muscularis propria. T3 disease invades the perirectal fat. T4 disease extends beyond the mesorectal fascia to directly invade other structures.

T1 and T2 diseases can be difficult to distinguish at MR. The hallmark of T3 disease is extension beyond the serosal surface of the rectum. Normally, at T2 MR the rectum is outlined by a thin black line. Such a line is seen from approximately 1 o'clock to 6 o'clock in the above case. Disruption of this line indicates tumor extension beyond the serosal surface of the rectum.

The distance between the tumor and the mesorectal fascia is an important data point for the surgeon as patients whose tumors extend to within 5 mm of the mesorectal fascia may benefit from neoadjuvant chemoradiation therapy prior to tumor removal.

The mesorectal fascia appears as a thin low-signal band at T2 MR which completely encircles the perirectal fat and is located approximately 2 to 3 cm away from the rectum. In the above image, normal mesorectal fascia is visible from approximately 1 o'clock to 8 o'clock.

Tumors that do not extend beyond the mesorectal fascia are usually removed via total mesorectal excision which includes resection of the tumor as well as the mesorectal fat. On the other hand, tumors that extend to within 5 mm of the mesorectal fascia are usually treated with chemoradiation first.

Question for Further Thought

1. In addition to measuring the distance between the tumor and the mesorectal fascia, what other measurement is helpful for preoperative planning?

Reporting Requirements

1. Describe if the tumor extends beyond the serosal surface of the rectum.
2. Report the distance between the tumor and the mesorectal fascia.
3. Report if the tumor invades adjacent organs.

What the Treating Physician Needs to Know

1. The distance between the tumor and the mesorectal fascia.

Answer

1. The distance between the tumor and the levator ani musculature as this distance can impact preoperative planning. The amount of normal rectum between the tumor and the levator ani musculature informs the surgeon's decision regarding whether a primary colonic anastomosis should be performed. For very low tumors, there may not be enough normal distal rectum left to perform a primary anastomosis and the patient may be left with a colostomy.

REFERENCE

1. Iafrate F, Laghi A, Paolantonio P, et al. Preoperative staging of rectal cancer with MR imaging: correlation with surgical and histopathologic findings. Radiographics 2006;26:701-714.

CLINICAL HISTORY *25-year-old woman with history of familial adenomatous polyposis (FAP) syndrome.*

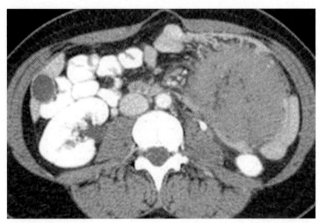

FIGURE 3.22A

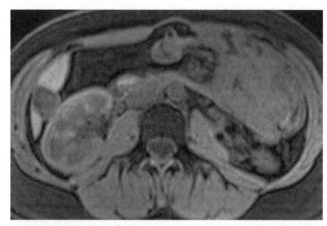

FIGURE 3.22B

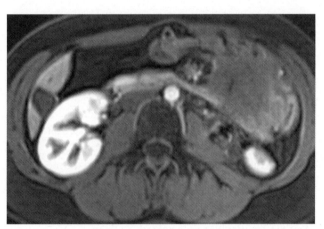

FIGURE 3.22C

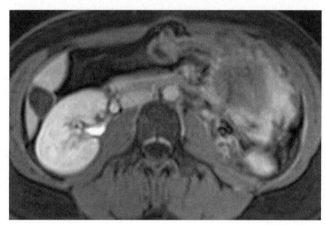

FIGURE 3.22D

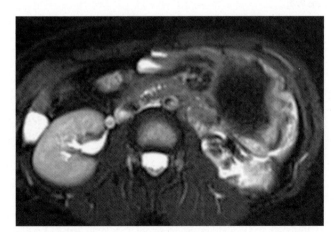

FIGURE 3.22E

FINDINGS CT image (A) demonstrates a large soft-tissue mass centered in the small bowel mesentery resulting in tethering and distortion of small bowel loops as well as left-sided hydronephrosis with a stent visible in the left ureter. T1-weighted MR imaging (B, precontrast; C 20-second delay [arterial phase]; and D, 3-minute delay) demonstrates heterogeneous, delayed hyperenhancement. The mass is primarily dark at T2-weighted imaging (E) (contrast agent: Gd-BOPTA [MultiHance; Bracco Diagnostics, Milan, Italy]).

DIFFERENTIAL DIAGNOSIS Carcinoid tumor, desmoid tumor, lymphoma.

DIAGNOSIS Desmoid tumor.

DISCUSSION Desmoid tumors are composed of fibroblasts. These tumors most frequently involve the small bowel mesentery or the anterior abdominal wall where they may occur at surgical scar sites. Though histologically benign, these infiltrative tumors may result in significant morbidity or mortality due to involvement of bowel loops, ureters, and/or blood vessels.

Desmoid tumors are most commonly sporadic. A minority of desmoid tumors occur in individuals with FAP. About 9% to 18% of patients with FAP develop desmoid tumors.

At CT, these tumors often appear as an enhancing, soft-tissue mesenteric mass. At MR, the appearance of these tumors is variable with, for example, T2 signal ranging from hypo- to hyperintense depending on the cellularity of the tumor. T1 signal may be hypo- to isointense with respect to muscle. A variety of enhancement patterns have been described ranging from no enhancement to homogeneous or heterogeneous enhancement.

Clinical history was key to making the correct diagnosis in the above case given the known association of FAP with desmoid tumors. Carcinoid tumors, unlike desmoid tumors, frequently calcify and may be associated with hepatic metastases. Additional sites of lymphadenopathy would be expected in a patient with mesenteric lymphoma.

Questions for Further Thought

1. What is the usual management of desmoid tumors?
2. Name other tumors associated with FAP.

Reporting Responsibilities

1. Describe the size and location of the mass.
2. Describe any complications such as bowel or ureteral obstruction.

What the Treating Physician Needs to Know

1. That a mesenteric or abdominal wall solid mass is most likely a desmoid tumor in a patient with FAP.

Answers

1. Management may include nonsteroidal anti-inflammatory drugs and antiestrogen medications. These tumors have a high rate of recurrence following resection.
2. FAP is an autosomal-dominant colorectal cancer syndrome. Given the near 100% likelihood of developing colon cancer by age 35 to 40, FAP patients usually undergo prophylactic colectomy. Patients may also develop upper gastrointestinal tract polyps. Gardner syndrome is a subdivision of FAP and includes osteomas, desmoid tumors, and soft-tissue tumors. Turcot syndrome is another subdivision of FAP and is associated with central nervous system tumors and desmoid tumors.

REFERENCES

1. Azizi L, Balu M, Belkacem A, Lewin M et al. MR feature of mesenteric desmoid tumors in familial adenomatous polyposis. Am J Roentgenol 2005;184:1128-1135.
2. Galiatsatos P, Foulkes WD. Familial adenomatous polyposis. Am J Gastroenterol 2006;101:385-398.